FOOD SAFETY ISSUES

Terrorist Threats to Food

Guidance for Establishing and Strengthening Prevention and Response Systems

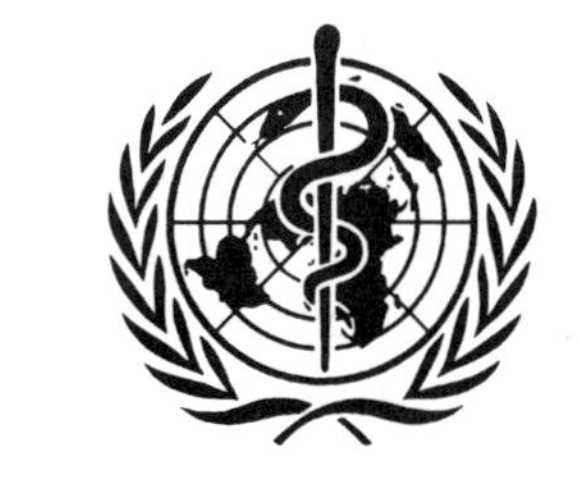

FOOD SAFETY DEPARTMENT
WORLD HEALTH ORGANIZATION

WHO Library Cataloguing-in-Publication Data

World Health Organization.
Terrorist threats to food : guidance for establishing and strengthening prevention and response systems.

(Food safety issues)

1.Food contamination - prevention and control   2.Food industry - standards
3.Terrorism - prevention and control 4.Biological warfare - prevention and control 5.
Disease outbreaks - prevention and control 6.Guidelines I.Title II.Series.

ISBN 92 4 154584 4   NLM classification: WA 701)

Food Safety Department
World Health Organization
Fax: +41 22 791 48 07
E.Mail: foodsafety@who.int
http://www.who.int/fsf

Terrorist Threats to Food: Guidance for Establishing and Strengthening Prevention and Response Systems

Contents

Executive Summary 1

1 Introduction 2

1.1   Purpose 2

1.2   Definitions and scope 3

1.3   Food as a vehicle for terrorist acts 3

1.4   Comparative risks of food and other media as vehicles for terrorist threats 5

1.5   Potential effects of food terrorism 5

    1.5.1   Illness and death 5
    1.5.2   Economic and trade effects 5
    1.5.3   Impact on public health services 6
    1.5.4   Social and political implications 7

1.6   Chemical and biological agents and radionuclear materials that could be used in food terrorism 7

1.7   Establishing and strengthening national prevention and response systems 7

1.8   Setting priorities 9

2 Prevention 10

2.1   Introduction 10

2.2   Existing systems 10

2.3   Strengthening food safety management programmes 11

2.4   Prevention and response systems in the food industry 12

    2.4.1   The role of the food industry 12
    2.4.2   Agricultural production and harvesting 13
    2.4.3   Processing and manufacture 13
    2.4.4   Storage and transport 14
    2.4.5   Wholesale and retail distribution 14
    2.4.6   Food service 15
    2.4.7   Tracing systems and market recalls 15
    2.4.8   Monitoring 15

2.5   Reducing access to chemical and biological agents and radionuclear materials 16

2.6   Prevention at points of entry 16

2.7   Useful source material 16

3 Surveillance, Preparedness and Response 18

    3.1   Introduction 18

    3.2   Surveillance 18

        3.2.1   Existing surveillance systems 18
        3.2.2   Strengthening existing surveillance systems for food safety 19
        3.2.3   Investigation of suspected food safety emergencies 20

    3.3   Preparedness 21

        3.3.1   Principles 21
        3.3.2   Assessing vulnerability 22

    3.4   Response 24

        3.4.1   Existing emergency response systems 24
        3.4.2   Strengthening existing emergency response systems for food safety 24
        3.4.3   Consequences of a food safety emergency 25
        3.4.4   Communication 27
        3.4.5   Launching the response 28

4 The Role of the World Health Organization 29

    4.1   International response to food safety emergencies, including food terrorism 29

    4.2   The World Health Organization 29

    4.3   International Health Regulations (IHR) 30

    4.4   Coordination of global outbreak alert and responses 31

        4.4.1   Outbreak alert mechanisms 31
        4.4.2   Global Outbreak Alert and Response Network 31
        4.4.3   Outbreak response 31

    4.5   Strengthening international systems to meet the threat of food terrorism 32

        4.5.1   Other existing WHO programmes relevant to food emergencies, including food terrorism 32
        4.5.2   Other international organizations relevant to food safety 34
        4.5.3   Coordination and strengthening of international strategies and activities that address food safety emergencies, including deliberate contamination of food 35

Appendix - Specific Measures for Consideration by the Food Industry 36

Executive Summary

The malicious contamination of food for terrorist purposes is a real and current threat, and deliberate contamination of food at one location could have global public health implications. This document responds to increasing concern in Member States that chemical, biological or radionuclear agents might be used deliberately to harm civilian populations and that food might be a vehicle for disseminating such agents. The Fifty-fifth World Health Assembly (May 2002) also expressed serious concern about such threats and requested the Organization to provide tools and support to Member States to increase the capacity of national health systems to respond.

Outbreaks of both unintentional and deliberate foodborne disease can be managed by the same mechanisms. Sensible precautions, coupled with strong surveillance and response capacity, constitute the most efficient and effective way of countering all such emergencies, including food terrorism. This document provides guidance to Member States for integrating consideration of deliberate acts of food sabotage into existing programmes for controlling the production of safe food. It also provides guidance on strengthening existing communicable disease control systems to ensure that surveillance, preparedness and response systems are sufficiently sensitive to meet the threat of any food safety emergency. Establishment and strengthening of such systems and programmes will both increase Member States' capacity to reduce the increasing burden of foodborne illness and help them to address the threat of food terrorism. The activities undertaken by Member States must be proportional to the size of the threat, and resources must be allocated on a priority basis.

Prevention, although never completely effective, is the first line of defence. The key to preventing food terrorism is establishment and enhancement of existing food safety management programmes and implementation of reasonable security measures. Prevention is best achieved through a cooperative effort between government and industry, given that the primary means for minimizing food risks lie with the food industry. This document provides guidance for working with industry, and specific measures for consideration by the industry are provided.

Member States require alert, preparedness and response systems that are capable of minimizing any risks to public health from real or threatened food terrorism. This document provides policy advice on strengthening existing emergency alert and response systems by improving links with all the relevant agencies and with the food industry. This multi-stakeholder approach will strengthen disease outbreak surveillance, investigation capacity, preparedness planning, effective communication and response.

The role of the World Health Organization (WHO) is to provide advice on strengthening of national systems to respond to food terrorism. WHO is also in a unique position to coordinate existing international systems for public health disease surveillance and emergency response, which could be expanded to include considerations of food terrorism. This document complements other guides and advice developed by WHO, the Food and Agriculture Organization of the United Nations (FAO) and other international agencies related to the threat of terrorist acts with chemical, biological or radionuclear agents.

Terrorist Threats to Food:

Guidance for Establishing and Strengthening Prevention and Response Systems

1. Introduction

Threats from terrorists, criminals and other anti-social groups who target the safety of the food supply are already a reality. During the past two decades, WHO Member States have expressed concern about the possibility that chemical and biological agents and radionuclear materials might deliberately be used to harm civilian populations. In recent months, the health ministries of several countries have increased their state of alert for intentional malevolent use of agents that may be spread through air, water or food.

On 18 May 2002, the Fifty-fifth World Health Assembly adopted a resolution (WHA 55.16) which expressed serious concern about threats against civilian populations by deliberate use of biological, chemical or radionuclear agents. It noted that such agents can be disseminated via food and requested the Director-General to provide tools and support to Member States, particularly developing countries, in strengthening their national systems. It also requested WHO to continue to issue international guidance and technical information on recommended public health measures to deal with deliberate use of chemical, biological or radionuclear agents to cause harm. In response, WHO has prepared these guidelines, intended primarily for policy-makers in national governments with responsibility for ensuring food safety, to assist them in incorporating considerations of food terrorism into existing systems for food safety.

Deliberate release of a chemical, biological or radionuclear agent could potentially cause severe harm and pose a huge burden on public health systems. Such a release would probably initially be considered as a natural or unintentional event. The Organization's traditional role has been to provide advice and support for strengthening food safety management programmes and public health disease alert and response systems at all levels. However, such systems need to be expanded to specifically address diseases that may be caused deliberately.

All Member States must have basic systems to prevent or deter deliberate contamination of their food supplies and, if attacked, to respond rapidly to minimize the health, economic and other effects of such contamination. However, counterterrorism should be seen as only one aspect of a broader, comprehensive food safety programme, in national and global contexts. WHO and a number of Member States have addressed this issue with strategies to reduce the increasing burden of foodborne illness. The WHO Global Strategy for Food Safety, endorsed in January 2002 by the WHO Executive Board, comprises a preventive approach to food safety, with increased surveillance and more rapid response to outbreaks of foodborne illness. This approach could substantially expand the abilities of Member States to protect the safety of their food supplies against natural and accidental threats and provides a framework for addressing terrorist threats to food.

1.1   *Purpose*

The purpose of this document is to provide policy guidance to Member States for integrating consideration of deliberate acts of sabotage of food into existing prevention and response programmes. Establishing and strengthening systems to address food terrorism, including disease outbreak surveillance and investigation, precautionary measures and emergency response systems, will give them a basic capacity to prevent and manage food safety emergencies, including food sabotage. This document also supports strengthening of programmes that underlie food production, processing and preparation to respond to food terrorism.

This document also describes the role of WHO, with its public health mandate, in responding to food safety emergencies of significance to international public health, which include food terrorist threats, and in providing assistance to Member States if their capacity to deal with such incidents is overwhelmed.

1.2   Definitions and scope

Food terrorism is defined as an act or threat of deliberate contamination of food for human consumption with chemical, biological or radionuclear agents for the purpose of causing injury or death to civilian populations and/or disrupting social, economic or political stability. The chemical agents in question are man-made or natural toxins, and the biological agents referred to are communicably infectious or non-infectious pathogenic microorganisms, including viruses, bacteria and parasites. Radionuclear agents are defined in this context as radioactive chemicals capable of causing injury when present at unacceptable levels. This document covers all food and includes water used in the preparation of food, as well as bottled water. However, water supply is not included in this document.

This document focuses on terrorist acts by non-State entities against governments, organizations and civilian populations and does not deal with acts of war perpetrated by one nation against another with chemical, radionuclear or biological weapons. It includes consideration of all means by which individuals seeking personal revenge or gain might deliberately contaminate food, including local acts of sabotage. Terrorist threats to animal or plant health or to the availability of food in sufficient quantity and variety to meet the nutritional needs of a population are not addressed.

A number of conventions prohibit the signatories from using biological, chemical or radionuclear weapons of mass destruction[1]. The objective of use of such agents by terrorists against a civilian population is essentially the same as that of their use in warfare against military targets: to cause widespread incapacitation and injury and to effect terror and panic. Civilian populations are usually more vulnerable than military personnel to chemical, biological or radionuclear weapons because they are of all ages and health status, whereas military personnel are generally healthy adults. Furthermore, the latter are usually prepared for attack by training and in many cases protected by immunization, prophylactics and protective clothing and devices. The potential agents and circumstances of terrorist attacks in civilian settings are more diverse than those directed at military personnel. As a result, rapid diagnosis and appropriate, readily available treatment may be difficult to assure. Because of this diversity the agents used by terrorists may be more readily obtainable than those used against military personnel.

1.3   Food as a vehicle for terrorist acts

There have been many instances where civilian food supplies have been sabotaged deliberately throughout recorded history, during military campaigns and, more recently, to terrorize or

---

[1] WHO. Public health response to biological and chemical weapons – WHO guidance – Projected second edition of Health aspects of chemical and biological weapons: report of the WHO group of consultants, Geneva 1970, republication issue for restricted distribution, November 2001.

otherwise intimidate civilian populations[2]. Deliberate contamination of food by chemical, biological or radionuclear agents can occur at any vulnerable point along the food chain, from farm to table, depending on both the food and the agent. For example, in 1984, members of a religious cult contaminated salad bars in the USA with *Salmonella typhimurium*, causing 751 cases of salmonellosis. The attack appeared to be a trial run for a more extensive attack intended to disrupt local elections. The cult was also in possession of strains of the causative organism of typhoid fever, a severe invasive illness[3]. In 1996, a disgruntled laboratory worker deliberately infected food to be consumed by colleagues with *Shigella dysenteria* type 2, causing illness in 12 people. Although few incidents or threats of deliberate contamination of food with chemical, biological or radionuclear agents on a massive scale have been documented, it is prudent to consider basic countermeasures.

The potential impact on human health of deliberate sabotage of food can be estimated by extrapolation from the many documented examples of unintentional outbreaks of foodborne disease. The largest, best-documented incidents include an outbreak of *S. typhimurium* infection in 1985, affecting 170 000 people, caused by contamination of pasteurized milk from a dairy plant in the USA[4]. An outbreak of hepatitis A associated with consumption of clams in Shanghai, China, in 1991 affected nearly 300 000 people and may be the largest foodborne disease incident in history[5]. In 1994, an outbreak of *S. enteritidis* infection from contaminated pasteurized liquid ice cream that was transported as a pre-mix in tanker trucks caused illness in 224 000 people in 41 states in the USA[6]. In 1996, about 8 000 children in Japan became ill, including some deaths, with *Escherichia coli* O157:H7 infection from contaminated radish sprouts served in school lunches[7].

Episodes of foodborne illness caused by chemicals have also been reported in the published literature. The chemicals that can contaminate food include pesticides, mycotoxins, heavy metals and other acutely toxic chemicals such as cyanide. In perhaps one of the most deadly incidents, over 800 people died and about 20 000 were injured, many permanently, by a chemical agent present in cooking oil sold in Spain in 1981[8]. In 1985, 1 373 people in the USA reported becoming ill after eating watermelon grown in soil treated with aldicarb[9].

Contamination of food in one country can also have a significant effect on health in other parts of the world. In 1989, staphylococcal food poisoning in the USA was associated with eating mushrooms that had been canned in China[10]. Outbreaks of cyclosporiasis in the USA in 1996

---

[2] Khan A. S., Swerdlow D. L., Juranek D. D. Precautions against biological and chemical terrorism directed at food and water supplies. Public Health Rep 2001;116:3–14.

[3] Torok T., Tauxe R. V., Wise R. P., et al. A large community outbreak of *Salmonella* caused by intentional contamination of restaurant salad bars. J Am Med Assoc 1997;278:389–95.

[4] Ryan C. A., Nickels M. K., Hargrett-Bean N. T., et al. Massive outbreak of antimicrobial-resistant salmonellosis traced to pasteurised milk. J Am Med Assoc 1987;258:3269–74.

[5] Halliday M. L., et al. An epidemic of hepatitis A attributable to the ingestion of raw clams in Shanghai, China. J Infect Dis 1991;164:852–9.

[6] Hennesy T. W., Hedberg C. W., Slutsker L., et al. A national outbreak of *Salmonella enteritides* infections from ice cream. New Engl J Med 1996; 334:1281–6.

[7] Mermin J. H., Griffin P. M. Invited commentary: public health crisis in crisis-outbreaks of *Escherichia coli* O157:H7 in Japan. Am J Epidemiol 1999;150:797–803.

[8] WHO Regional Office for Europe. Toxic oil syndrome: Mass food poisoning in Spain. Report of a WHO meeting, Madrid, 21–25 May 1983, Copenhagen: WHO Regional Office for Europe 1984.

[9] Green M. A., Heumann M. A., Wehr H. M., et al. An outbreak of watermelon-borne pesticide toxicity. Am J Public Health 1987;77:1431–4.

[10] Levine W. C., Bennet R. W., Choy Y., et al. Staphylococcal food poisoning caused by imported canned mushrooms. J Infect Dis 1996;173:1263–7.

and 1997 were linked to consumption of Guatemalan raspberries[11]. Many similar outbreaks have been reported in the literature.

1.4   Comparative risks of food and other media as vehicles for terrorist threats

Certain chemical and biological agents and radionuclear materials can be disseminated as small-particle aerosols or volatile liquids for the purposes of an airborne attack on civilian populations. Such formulations have already been made as weapons for tactical or strategic use on the battlefield. This mode of attack is, however, subject to major uncertainties, as air movements, conditions in enclosed spaces, stability of the agent, particle size and dose needed to achieve an effect. Similarly, effective deliberate contamination of reticulated water supplies presents other challenges and limitations.

Deliberate contamination of food might, in some regards, be easier to control than attacks through air or water. The safety of food is closely controlled in many developed countries, both by the government and the private sector. Food safety infrastructures offer a means for preventing and mitigating sabotage of the food supply. The dietary diversity available in many developed countries also reduces the likelihood that the entire food supply would be contaminated and would tend to dilute potential health effects. In addition, international food safety initiatives and enhanced disease surveillance and response activities can be developed for preventing and responding quickly to food terrorism. On the other hand, food is also the most vulnerable to intentional contamination by debilitating or lethal agents. The diversity of sources of foods, including the global market, makes prevention difficult, if not impossible. At the same time, many developing countries lack basic food safety infrastructures and are vulnerable to deliberate acts of sabotage.

1.5   Potential effects of food terrorism

1.5.1   Illness and death

The potential impact of contaminated food on human health from deliberate acts of sabotage can be inferred from reports of unintended foodborne disease outbreaks, as outlined above. If an unintentional outbreak from one food, such as clams, can affect 300 000 individuals, a concerted, deliberate attack could be devastating, especially if a more dangerous chemical, biological or radionuclear agent was used. Clearly, the potential health effects of a terrorist attack must be taken seriously by the health community and by those responsible for assessing and countering terrorist threats.

1.5.2   Economic and trade effects

Deliberate contamination of food may also have enormous economic implications, even if the episode is relatively minor. In fact, economic disruption may be a primary motive for a deliberate act, targeting a product, a manufacturer, an industry or a country. Mass casualties are not required to achieve widespread economic loss and disruption of trade. Extortion threats directed at specific organizations, particularly those in the commercial sector, are commoner than is generally believed.

In an effort to damage Israel's economy in 1978, citrus fruit exported to several European countries was contaminated with mercury, which led to significant trade disruption. The alleged

---

[11] Herwaldt B. L., Ackers M-L. Cyclospora working group. An outbreak in 1996 of cyclosporiasis associated with imported raspberries. New Engl J Med 1997;336:1548–56.

contamination of Chilean grapes with cyanide in 1989 led to the recall of all Chilean fruit from Canada and the USA, and the publicity surrounding this incident resulted in a boycott by American consumers. The resulting damage amounted to several hundred million dollars and more than 100 growers and shippers went bankrupt[12]. In 1998, a company in the USA recalled 14 million kilograms of frankfurters and luncheon meats potentially contaminated with *Listeria*. The parent company closed the plant and estimated their total cost to be US$50–70 million[13]. An outbreak of *E. coli* O157:H7 infection in the USA in 1997 resulted in the recall of 11 million kilograms of ground beef[14].

The crisis in Belgium in which dioxin-contaminated meat and dairy products were recalled around the world demonstrates not only the extensive costs to individual countries, but also the extent of disruption of global trade that can be caused by this type of incident. Consumer concern about consumption of meat potentially affected by the agent responsible for bovine spongiform encephalopathy and linked to the new variant Creutzfeldt-Jakob disease is still disrupting trade world-wide, with costs yet to be calculated and a significant long-term impact on meat production in many countries. The outbreak of foot-and-mouth disease in the United Kingdom in 2000 is another example of a major economic and trade dislocation.

Thus, deliberate sabotage of food could have serious economic and trade repercussions. Industries in many sectors could be put out of business, and countries could experience severe economic and trade disruption. In less developed countries, the economic consequences of a terrorist act on food could also affect development and exacerbate poverty as well as food availability.

1.5.3   Impact on public health services

Foodborne illness, whether intentional or otherwise, can also paralyse public health services. The 1995 attack with nerve gas in on commuters on the Tokyo subway system, while not foodborne, clearly illustrates the effects of a coordinated terrorist attack on an unsuspecting population. This highly publicised attack caused the deaths of 12 people and led 5 000 people to seek medical care. The response to the incident was prompt and massive, with 131 ambulances and 1 364 emergency technicians dispatched and 688 people transported to hospital by emergency medical and fire services. More that 4 000 people found their own way to hospitals and doctors[15].

Many countries do not have the capacity to respond to such massive emergencies. The public health service facilities for coping with these types of emergencies and for providing continuing care may be strained to the limit. While many countries have some form of emergency response plan, they usually do not include consideration of food safety. This gap in preparedness could lead to misdiagnosis, incorrect laboratory investigations and failure to identify and detain affected food. This would weaken or even preclude an effective response to a food sabotage incident.

---

[12] Root-Bernstein R. S. Infectious terrorism. Atlantic Monthly May 1991.

[13] Centers for Disease Control and Prevention. Update: multi-state outbreak of listeriosis – United States, 1998–1999. Morbid Mortal Wkly Rep 1999;47:1117–8.

[14] Centers for Disease Control and Prevention. *Escherichia coli* O157:H7 infections associated with eating a nationally distributed commercial brand of frozen ground beef patties and hamburgers: Colorado, 1997. Mortal Morbid Wkly Rep 1997;46:77–8.

[15] Okumura T. et al. Tokyo subway Sarin attack: disaster management. Part 2: hospital response. Academic Emergency Medicine, 1998, 5:681-624

1.5.4 Social and political implications

Terrorists may have a variety of motives, from revenge to political destabilization. They may target the civilian population to create panic and threaten civil order. As the response to mailing of envelopes containing *Bacillus anthracis* in the USA showed, limited dissemination of biological agents by simple means, causing few cases of illness, can cause considerable disruption and public anxiety[16]. Fear and anxiety may contribute to reduced confidence in the political system and government, and may therefore result in political destabilization. When the effects are economic and lead to loss of income for some sectors of society, the political impact can be exacerbated. Finally, while contamination of the entire food supply is unlikely, pre-existing food shortages could be worsened by deliberate contamination, again with an impact on political and social stability.

1.6 Chemical and biological agents and radionuclear materials that could be used in food terrorism

Access to chemical and biological agents and radionuclear materials that have been developed as weapons is limited, and their production and stockpiling are controlled under specific treaties and agreements[17]. However, more readily available toxic chemicals, including pesticides, heavy metals and industrial chemicals as well as a plethora of naturally occurring microbiological pathogens, could be used as agents in terrorist threats to food. Their effective use would depend on their potential impact on human health, the food used for their dissemination and the point of introduction into the food chain. The agents used could have acute effects, resulting in death, paralysis or vomiting, or long-term consequences, such as fetal abnormalities and increased rates of chronic illness such as cancer. Therefore, the latency period before any harm is manifested also needs to be considered.

The Centers for Disease Control and Prevention (CDC) in the USA have issued a list of critical biological agents as a part of their strategic plan for preparedness for terrorist incidents[18], but the list does not include most chemical agents. Their approach, which consists of examining the consequences of an attack, can be adapted for chemical and radionuclear agents. While this approach is useful for an initial analysis of vulnerability, the risk posed by a specific agent in a specific food may have to be examined on a case-by-case basis. Various parameters, such as the fate of an agent under specific conditions, must be assessed to estimate the risk in particular situations. The point of introduction of an agent into the food chain must also be considered to ensure that the risk assessment remains valid and the response is appropriate to the threat.

1.7 Establishing and strengthening national prevention and response systems

Most countries have some form of emergency response system in place to respond to catastrophic incidents such as earthquakes, floods or disease outbreaks that threaten the health of the population. However, these response systems rarely include consideration of terrorism and even more rarely include consideration of food as a vehicle for delivering harmful agents. Such gaps in the capacity to prevent and respond to the broadest range of food safety

---

[16] Sobel J., Khan A. S., Swerdlow K. L. Threat of biological terrorist attack on the US food supply: the CDC perspective. Lancet 2002; 359:874-880.

[17] WHO. Public health response to biological and chemical weapons – WHO guidance – Projected second edition of health aspects of chemical and biological weapons: report of the WHO group of consultants, Geneva 1970, republication issue for restricted distribution, November 2001.

[18] Centres for Disease Control and Prevention. Biological and chemical terrorism: strategic plan for preparedness and response – recommendations of the CDC strategic planning workgroup. Morb Mortal Wkly Rep 2000; 49:1–14.

emergencies must be closed to ensure effective responses. Each Member State should consider its own needs and priorities in respect of food terrorism to ensure that its measures are proportional to its other public health priorities.

The two major strategies for countering the threat of food sabotage are prevention and response, including preparedness. Chapter 2 outlines the preventive aspects that can be incorporated into food safety programmes to meet the new threat of food sabotage and to assist governments in working with the food industry to strengthen food safety and security during production, processing and preparation. The food safety systems and infrastructure in place in many countries to ensure the safety of the food supply, and thus reduce the burden of foodborne illness, include safety management programmes for food production and processing. These could be modified relatively simply to incorporate basic considerations to prevent food sabotage. The food industry has the primary responsibility for assuring the safety of the food they produce, and government agencies, working with the private sector, have regulatory and advisory responsibility in promoting safe food measures by industry, including good agricultural and good manufacturing practices.

Chapter 3 addresses the surveillance, preparedness and response elements specific to food safety, to facilitate their inclusion in existing national emergency response plans and to achieve balance between threats to food safety and other threats. Plans to respond to food safety emergencies should complement, not replace, other critical activities, and resources should be allocated on the basis of the nature and likelihood of such threats. Vulnerability should be assessed in order to evaluate the most likely risks from food sabotage and set priorities for risk management. Increased attention must be paid to risk communication, to reduce the likelihood of panic and loss of public confidence.

For the purpose of this document, response includes all measures to identify, contain and minimize the impact of a food terrorist incident. Once a terrorist attack is known or suspected to have occurred, it is vital that the response to the situation be speedy and effective. Plans to mitigate the effects of sabotage of the food supply should thus be incorporated within existing emergency response systems. Separate systems would be wasteful of resources, especially as there are many common elements of response to natural or accidental incidents that may threaten public health. Nevertheless, a system for responding to food sabotage possesses some unique aspects. For example, national emergency plans should incorporate laboratory capacity for analysing uncommon agents in food. It should also have closer links with food tracing and recall systems. The aspects specific to food are outlined in this document.

In Chapter 4, the current activities of WHO in this regard and a proposal for strengthening collaboration to assure more effective alert and response systems for food terrorism are presented. With the globalization of the world's food supply, an attack on one country's food supply cannot be seen in isolation. Food is a major item of trade for many countries; furthermore, most countries, including developing countries, are both importers and exporters of food. Globalization of the world's media assures that any terrorist attack on a nation's food supply will receive intense, and perhaps disproportionate, attention. Consequently, the response to a terrorist threat to food will require collaboration with United Nations specialized agencies such as WHO and FAO, and possibly other international organizations.

Developing countries have various levels of food safety infrastructure and alert and emergency response systems, and they may require strengthening. Incomplete systems increase vulnerability to foodborne disease. The guidelines given in this document should be considered in the context of WHO's existing mechanism for establishing and strengthening national infrastructures for food safety.

1.8   Setting priorities

Member States face competing demands on their resources, and terrorist threats, including the possibility of food terrorism, must be balanced against other priorities. Assessment at this level may include consideration of the means and will to terrorize the civilian population and the potential social, political and economic consequences of such threats. The resources allocated to the public health sector must be commensurate with the magnitude and likelihood of threat. However, as a matter of prudence, all countries should put in place basic contingency plans for food safety emergencies.

Priority setting in the public health sector must include assessment of other health problems in relation to food terrorism. Once a decision is taken to increase the capacity of the national system to respond to food terrorist threats, the most vulnerable foods and food processes should be identified, including:

- the most readily accessible food processes;

- foods that are most vulnerable to undetected tampering;

- foods that are the most widely disseminated or spread; and

- the least supervised food production areas and processes.

2. Prevention

2.1 Introduction

As in all health and safety considerations, prevention is the most desirable option. In the context of food terrorism, prevention means preventing the sabotage of food during production, processing, distribution and preparation. While safeguarding chemical, biological or radionuclear agents before they can be used is important, this chapter does not focus on the individual agents that could be used to contaminate food. This chapter presents various approaches for protecting food production systems to reduce the likelihood and impact of a terrorist attack.

The key to preventing food terrorism is enhancing existing food safety programmes and implementing reasonable security measures on the basis of assessments of vulnerability. The deliberate introduction of a chemical, biological or radionuclear agent into food during production, processing, distribution or preparation of food may be a relatively new threat for industries and governments. As many production methods and food safety programmes are proprietary, the food industry has both the responsibility and the capacity to reduce the likelihood of deliberate contamination of food, from the raw materials to product distribution. Governments should support industry in strengthening existing food safety management systems, to include consideration of deliberate contamination. Governments also have a role in promoting preventive food safety, through established voluntary and regulatory mechanisms[19].

2.2 Existing systems

Many governments have, or are developing, food safety infrastructures to ensure that food produced for domestic consumption meets acceptable safety criteria and that food produced for export meets international food safety standards. Strengthening national food safety programmes requires that national policies and resources to support the infrastructure are in place and that food legislation, food monitoring and surveillance, food inspection, foodborne disease surveillance, education and training are adequate and up to date. Proactive risk analysis can reduce vulnerability in the same way as analysis of the risks of inadvertent contamination. The resources allocated need to be proportional to the likelihood of the threat, the magnitude and severity of the consequences and the vulnerability of the system. The possibility of intentional contamination needs to be an integral part of safety considerations, and measures to prevent sabotage should augment, not replace, other activities. Typical food safety management programmes within the food industry include good agricultural practice, good manufacturing practice and 'hazard analysis and critical control point' (HACCP) and HACCP-based systems.

As with other aspects of food safety programmes, priorities for action are determined by an analysis of the hazards specific for each food operation. The risk should be analysed for each link in the food chain, taking into consideration other country-specific issues, such as the availability of chemical, biological or radionuclear agents. Consideration of the threats at each link may include issues such as vulnerability to sabotage, opportunity for the introduction of an agent and capacity to monitor deliberate contamination and to trace and recall suspect products. This approach will enable effective prevention by focusing efforts and resources on the most important threats.

Food can be contaminated deliberately by chemical, biological or radionuclear agents at any point in the food chain (see Figure 1). Food safety management programmes offer opportunities

---

[19] WHO. Guidelines for strengthening a national food safety programme. WHO/FNU/FOS/96.2. Geneva, 1996.

for the prevention, detection and control of food sabotage. Understanding the relationships between the production system, ingredients, people, utensils, equipment and machinery can help in identifying where critical failures of the system might occur. Methods of sabotage and the extent of a threat might be identified as a part of this analysis and would provide the basis for a risk analysis.

Figure 1. General overview of the typical food chain

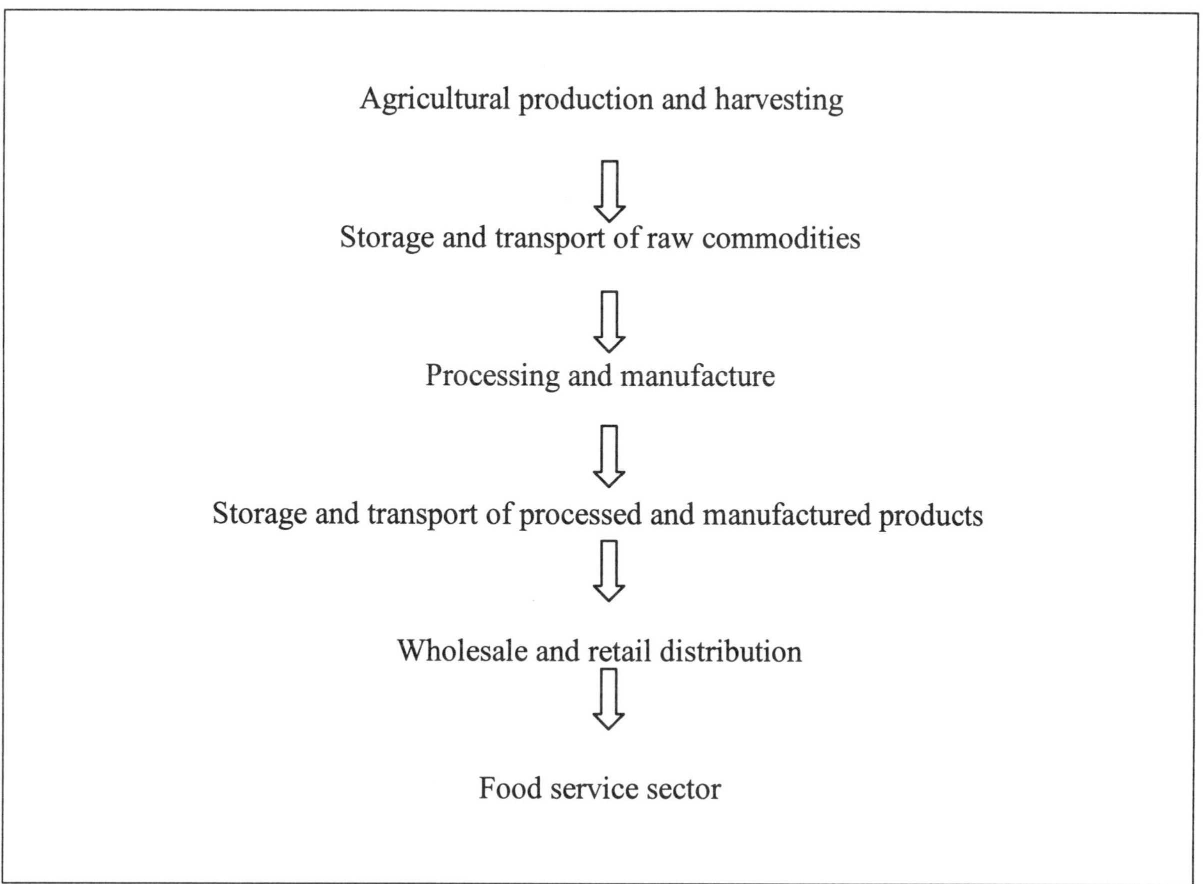

2.3   Strengthening food safety management programmes

Governments should work with industry to incorporate considerations of food terrorism into food safety management programmes. Not all countries have the infrastructure needed to assist industry, especially small, less developed businesses, to approach food production, processing and preparation on the basis of food safety management principles. In the absence of such infrastructure, it may be difficult to prevent deliberate contamination of the food supply. In such situations, systems for rapid detection of and response to food terrorism may also be poorly developed. Capacity building for such competence is vital for the prevention of both intentional and unintentional contamination of food. The generic actions taken by government to assist industry in this respect should include:

- cooperating with industry to develop protocols for assessing the vulnerability of individual food businesses, including assessments of the site, security and personnel, and potential ways in which food might be contaminated maliciously (see section 3.3.2);

- ensuring that food safety is addressed and controls are coordinated at all links of the food chain, including traceability and recall;

- cooperating with industry to strengthen the security of processes, people and products;

- providing industry with information on known or possible biological, chemical and radionuclear agents;

- cooperating with industry to develop, implement, review and test crisis management plans; and

- coordinating closely with industry in communicating with the public.

Prevention of terrorist attacks does not always require high technology or great expense. Increased awareness of the problem and enhanced vigilance are among the effective measures that can be taken. Awareness can be heightened by auditing food safety management programmes. In the event of an incident, information from early surveillance could be shared with the food industry to facilitate prompt action to address consumer concerns and contain and mitigate the threat.

2.4   Prevention and response systems in the food industry

2.4.1   The role of the food industry

The capacity to prevent deliberate sabotage of food lies mainly with the food industry and must be addressed throughout the food chain. Potential contamination with chemical and biological agents and radionuclear materials and interruption of food supplies need to be considered in assessments of food safety management programmes. Whether a food safety management programme is rudimentary or well developed, further elaboration should focus on the nature and extent of the threat. The response needs to be proportional to the identified threat.

Food production systems range from farms, with goods marketed to neighbouring communities, to large corporations with global production and distribution systems. Many foods, such as fish, meat, poultry, fruit and vegetables, are consumed with minimal processing. Others, such as cereal products and cooking oils, undergo considerable processing before reaching the consumer. The production system and the steps vulnerable to attack will therefore be different for each type of food. Often, it is the interfaces between components of the chain, where food changes hands, that are the most vulnerable to sabotage. The potential for intentional contamination of products is likely to increase as the point of contamination nears the points of production and distribution. However, the potential for greater individual morbidity or mortality usually increases as the agent is introduced closer to the point of consumption.

The Appendix to this document *Specific Measures for Consideration by the Food Industry* provides guidance to industry for strengthening food safety management programmes to prevent both inadvertent and intentional contamination of food with harmful agents. However, this Appendix is not meant to mandate action but to offer a spectrum of actions that could be considered by industry in a manner proportional to the perceived threat. Small and medium size industry will need to set priorities for implementation as resources permit.

Opportunities for deliberate contamination of food can be minimized by increasing the security of people and premises. All segments of the food industry could develop security and response plans for their establishments, proportional to the threat and their resources. Sources of raw materials and storage facilities and transport systems might have to be safeguarded. Access to all critical areas in production, processing, transport and storage could be controlled and documented to minimize opportunities for contamination.

Employers could consider screening their staff to ensure that their qualifications and background are compatible with their work and responsibilities. Sanitation, maintenance and inspection workers, who have access to critical areas, could also be vetted from a security perspective. All staff could be encouraged to report suspicious behaviour and activities to the appropriate authorities. However, such encouragement should be qualified to prevent false or unwarranted reports for the purpose of harassment.

2.4.2 Agricultural production and harvesting

Recent incidents of contamination of bovine feed with the causative agent of bovine spongiform encephalitis and contamination of poultry feed with dioxins illustrate the national and international effects that inadvertent contamination has had on human and animal health, consumer confidence and national economies. Many animal feed ingredients are important on the international market. Safety assurance systems could be included in the control of animal feed and feed ingredients. Security measures, such as control of access and tamper-resistant or tamper-evident systems, such as tape or wax seals, could be considered during manufacture, transport and storage. Mechanisms for tracing and recall of animal feeds and animal feed ingredients could be considered, where feasible.

Agricultural production areas vary from those of smallholdings to those of very large commercial farms and feedlots. While emphasis has heretofore been on production efficiency, recent programmes to promote good agricultural practice explicitly include concern for food safety. Agricultural production areas are vulnerable to deliberate contamination. Attention should be paid to possible substitution of pesticides with more toxic agents and contamination of irrigation water. Subsequent processing may include critical control points for the detection and control of inadvertent or deliberate contamination. As fruits and vegetables are consumed directly, with minimal processing, there are few critical control points for detection or removal of contamination. The many incidents of inadvertent contamination of meat, fish, poultry, and milk products with pathogenic microorganisms during production are clear indications of the vulnerability of these commodities.

The point of introduction of raw materials into the processing stream is a critical control point in most processing operations. Good agricultural practice (including use of HACCP-like systems) is being implemented in many primary production areas. Coupled with routine inspections, these can greatly reduce the likelihood of inadvertent or deliberate contamination. Certain harvesting practices, such as open-air drying, offer opportunities for deliberate contamination. Controlling access to and monitoring of agricultural production areas could be considered, particularly in response to known or likely threats. Sources of raw materials with secure operations could be used whenever possible. Since analysis for all possible threats is impossible, emphasis could be placed on determining deviations from normal characteristics. The potential for deliberate contamination could be considered in sampling and analysis of the final processed products. Appropriate follow-up, such as recall and tracing back for contamination, are necessary in the case of all deviations that may indicate contamination.

2.4.3 Processing and manufacture

The possibility of deliberate contamination must be included in food safety programmes for food processing and manufacture. The slaughterhouse stage in the food production chain can be vulnerable, particularly if it is not covered by food safety management programmes or comparable systems. The water used in food processing is an important consideration, particularly for minimally processed foods such as fruits and vegetables, where washing is often the only processing step. Approaches similar to those used those for drinking-water systems, including analysis, could be applied. It is important to prevent and respond to attacks on water for food industry use, as would be the case for drinking water supply. Protection and inspection of facilities, including water sources, are particularly important as they may be located some distance from the food processing plant. Air systems in processing plants could also be sources of inadvertent or deliberate contamination. In many food-processing systems, heat treatment is a critical control point for microbiological contaminants. From the point of view of deliberate contamination, the normal time and temperature treatments at these control points might not be adequate for all microbiological agents that could be used and would have little or no effect on reducing contamination by toxic chemicals.

Access to all critical areas and equipment, including storage areas and water and air systems, could be controlled and monitored. Closed systems are often perceived to be less vulnerable and are therefore often subject to less surveillance. However, they could be considered in assessing terrorist threats. Personal items, such as lunch containers, could be prohibited from critical areas.

2.4.4 Storage and transport

Even though storage facilities for raw agricultural commodities range from the open air to large elevators and the means of transport range from human portage to large ocean-going vessels, some precautions are generally applicable. Physical measures, such as fencing and locks, can be used to secure and prevent unauthorized access to storage facilities and transport containers. These could be supplemented with on-site security personnel, intrusion detectors and alarms. If resources permit, silent alarms linked to the appropriate authorities or remote-controlled television surveillance could be introduced. Tamper-resistant and tamper-evident packaging for larger lots as well as for single packages could be considered. All returned products could be carefully examined before reshipment.

International and domestic transport of food is being handled increasingly in containers, except in the case of bulk food shipments, in which the food commodity, such as grain, is loaded directly into the conveyance. Tamper-resistant or tamper-evident locks or seals on containers can be improvised from materials such as annotated tapes and waxes, which are widely available. Temperature controls and monitoring devices on refrigerated containers could be constructed to prevent unauthorized access.

2.4.5 Wholesale and retail distribution

While tamper-resistant and tamper-evident containers have proved to be extremely useful in reducing deliberate contamination, all such containers are vulnerable to individuals who know how to penetrate the protective measures. Controlled access and greater vigilance, including cameras and other types of surveillance, may be needed to increase security.

Bulk foods are particularly vulnerable to deliberate contamination in many markets. More secure containers for bulk foods and use of pre-packaged materials could be considered to prevent deliberate contamination. Wholesale and retail managers could use reliable suppliers. Substitution of sub-standard food products for products of greater value (counterfeiting) occurs in most parts of the world, and this activity has included use of false labels and replaced ingredients. In some cases the replaced ingredients were contaminated with toxic chemicals. The same approach could be used to distribute sabotaged products. Buyers should be suspicious of food being sold under unusual circumstances, such as at much lower prices than normal or outside normal distribution channels.

2.4.6 Food service

Food service operations have already been the target of criminal attacks. Condiments in open containers in restaurants and institutional settings are vulnerable to deliberate contamination. Increased monitoring of salad bars and other communal food displays may be necessary to deter deliberate contamination. Automatic dispensing equipment, including vending machines, may also be vulnerable to contamination. Consideration could be given to increased surveillance and additional tamper-resistant and tamper-evident devices.

As for inadvertent contamination, washing and cooking food adequately before consumption could be emphasized. Careful attention could be given to tamper-resistant or tamper-evident seals. When the integrity of a seal or a container is in doubt or the food product does not meet the usual expectations of quality, such as an abnormal appearance, odour or taste, it should not be purchased or consumed. If tampering is suspected, food service personnel could be encouraged and provided with a means of notifying (for example phone number on the label) the retailer or supplier and the appropriate public health and law enforcement authorities.

2.4.7 Tracing systems and market recalls

Many foods are produced at centralized facilities and distributed over large geographical areas, often globally. Contamination at such facilities can affect large numbers of people, and exposure may be widespread before the outbreak is detected. Rapid determination of the source of contamination and localization of the contaminated product can greatly reduce the number of casualties, by facilitating rapid removal of the contaminated products from the market. Withdrawal back to the point in the processing chain where the contamination occurred is essential for protecting the public from terrorist threats.

Tracing systems and market recalls are thus critical in responding to food contamination, whether deliberate or inadvertent. However, tracing systems for contaminated products are not always simple, as evidenced by the dioxin crisis in Belgium and several other food safety emergencies.

Many agriculture production systems are not suited to adopt mechanisms for recall. Raw agricultural products produced on small farms are usually co-mingled and combined with other co-mingled lots to form larger shipments. Thus, in most cases, it is difficult to identify the producer of a contaminated shipment. For raw materials, the extent of recall must depend on consideration of the resources required for tracing and market recall compared with the resources needed for analysis and other measures for determining safety at the critical control point of the processing stream.

2.4.8 Monitoring

Monitoring programmes can include a range of approaches, from careful visual examination to high technology in-line detection systems. As with inadvertent contamination, it is virtually impossible, both technically and economically, to carry out analyses for all agents all the time. In many cases, indicators of non-specific variations in product specifications raise concern. Resources for routine monitoring might therefore be appropriately allocated for specific products, processes and handling situations. Rapid follow-up is essential if variation in product specifications is seen that could indicate deliberate contamination. Public health officials could work closely with commercial and other private sector organizations, where possible, in developing appropriate monitoring programmes.

2.5 Reducing access to chemical and biological agents and radionuclear materials

Limiting access to chemical and biological agents and radionuclear materials that could be used to contaminate the food supply deliberately can contribute to counterterrorism. While some agents developed as weapons by military forces could be used to contaminate food, relatively common chemicals and pathogens may pose more significant threats to food. Highly toxic pesticides and industrial chemicals, including chemical waste, are available in most areas of the world. Pathogenic microbiological agents are present in clinical and other laboratories, including laboratories involved in food control. University-level knowledge of chemistry or microbiology is sometimes sufficient to make effective amounts of many agents. Radionuclear materials are widely available for medical research.

Guidance already exists on the safety and security of laboratory materials[20]. Governments and commercial organizations should increase the security of stores of toxic drugs, pesticides, radionuclear materials and other chemicals and immediately report any theft or other unauthorized diversion to the proper authorities. Greater effort should be made to control the availability of microbiological pathogens. It is critical that clinical, research and food control laboratories be aware of this potential and take appropriate security measures to minimize the risk that such materials are diverted.

The development, production and use of chemical and biological agents as weapons are covered by international and national laws and agreements. These are essential to protect the public against hostile release of such agents. WHO has developed advice to mitigate the consequences should such a release of this nature take place[21].

2.6 Prevention at points of entry

Quarantine and customs agencies contribute to preventing food safety emergencies by controlling the entry of contaminated food into importing countries. However, in most countries that rely significantly on imported food, it would be virtually impossible to inspect and analyse all shipments. Linkages must be set up between all food safety sectors, including the authorities in the country of origin, quarantine and customs officials, food importers, food safety agencies and state security authorities, in order to set priorities and to enhance inspection and monitoring.

2.7 Useful source material

All possible scenarios of food sabotage cannot be described in this document. Credible risks need to be considered at every point in the food chain to ensure the safety of the food produced. A number of useful documents prepared by certain Member States[22,23,24] and industries[25] offer

---

[20] WHO. Safety in health care laboratory. WHO/LAB/97.1. Geneva.

[21] WHO. Public health response to biological and chemical weapons – WHO guidance – Projected second edition of health aspects of chemical and biological weapons: report of the WHO group of consultants, Geneva 1970, republication issue for restricted distribution, November 2001.

[22] Canadian Food Inspection Agency. Notice to food processors and distributors, suggestions for improving security. www.inspection.gc.ca/english/ops/secur/protrae.shtml.

[23] Canadian Food Inspection Agency. Notice to food retailers, suggestions for improving security. www.inspection.gc.ca/english/ops/secur/retdete.shtml.

[24] Canadian Food Inspection Agency. Notice to livestock operations, suggestions for improving security. www.inspection.gc.ca/english/ops/secur/livebete.shtml-

examples and guidance for analysing risks in the production and processing of specific foods. The documents also provide advice and examples to the food industry for incorporating considerations of terrorist threats within existing food safety management programmes. Not all of these documents will be applicable in their entirety to smaller, developing businesses, but the general principles of assessing vulnerability apply across all businesses and sectors[26,27].

[25] Food and Drug Administration Center for Food Safety and Applied Nutrition. Food safety and security: operational risk management systems approach (ORM), November 2001. Washington DC: Department of Health and Social Security.

[26] Food and Drug Administration Center for Food Safety and Applied Nutrition. Guidance for industry, food producers, processors, transporters and retailers: food security preventive measures guidance, 2002, http://www.cfsan.fda.gov/~dms/secguid.html.

[27] Food and Drug Administration Center for Food Safety and Applied Nutrition. Guidance for industry, importers and filers: food security preventive measures guidance, 2002, http://www.cfsan.fda.gov/~dms/secguid2.html.

3. Surveillance, Preparedness and Response

3.1   Introduction

It is highly unlikely that acts of food terrorism can be completely prevented, and it is even more unlikely, if not impossible, to prevent hoaxes. Much of the scientific knowledge required to produce chemical and biological agents that could be used to contaminate food deliberately is in the public domain. However, sensible precautions coupled with effective surveillance, preparedness and response systems can do much to counter food terrorism. While most of the capacity to prevent food safety emergencies lies within the food industry, governments have a lead responsibility for detecting and responding to actual or threatened food terrorism incidents as well as other food safety emergencies. When suspected or adulterated food reaches the consumer, the potential consequences to public health, the economy and social or political stability must be managed by an effective, rapid emergency response system. Existing systems for surveillance, preparedness and emergency response need to be strengthened to increase their ability to address food terrorism.

Covert or overt acts of food terrorism must first be detected by surveillance and other alert systems, before a response can be activated. The response may include verification of a threat, including the cause of disease, management of the consequences by aiding the affected population, identification and removal of the food from sale and management of the social, political and economic consequences of the act. These activities may have be carried out concurrently. Rapid, effective management of the consequences of food terrorism must be based on well-planned links between the existing components of a national emergency response plan and those responsible for food terrorism.

This chapter briefly outlines the components of emergency surveillance, preparedness and response systems, focusing mainly on potential gaps with respect to food terrorism and suggesting ways of filling such gaps.

3.2   Surveillance

3.2.1   Existing surveillance systems

The main requirement for rapid detection of an epidemic is a surveillance system that is sensitive for identifying small clusters of illness. Such systems permit identification of all disease outbreaks, whether intentional or unintentional, but do not necessarily permit identification of the disease or its mode of transmission. Surveillance systems also provide information about the expected frequency and size of various disease outbreaks, thus providing a baseline for identifying unusual clusters that might herald a terrorist incident. Early detection of disease resulting from covert food terrorism depends on sensitive surveillance systems for communicable disease at local and national levels, with close cooperation and communication among clinicians, laboratories and public health professionals.

Many Member States maintain surveillance systems for communicable diseases, which are collaborative efforts based on passive or active surveillance systems and often include a requirement for mandatory reporting of specific diseases and the pathogens that cause them. These systems are not detailed here, as the focus of the document is to address the addition of food safety components to such systems.

3.2.2   Strengthening existing surveillance systems for food safety

Many existing surveillance systems may have the capacity to detect clusters of foodborne disease, provided the cluster is large enough and the effects severe enough to cause people to seek medical attention. However, as the focus of these systems is communicable diseases, their capacity to detect and investigate foodborne illness rapidly may require the addition of parameters specific for food and agents that can cause foodborne illness. Surveillance networks for communicable diseases can thus be extended to detect foodborne disease clusters by the addition of systems to collect and interpret the necessary data.

A number of Member States already maintain surveillance systems to detect and investigate foodborne disease. In many cases, such systems are passive and rely on reporting by laboratories or physicians. Statistical analysis of information from such systems can reveal unusual clustering of diseases by time or geographical area as compared with baseline values. Unfortunately, passive surveillance systems result in underreporting, because only a small fraction of ill people seek medical care or submit samples for laboratory analysis. Furthermore, laboratories sometimes test for only a fraction of disease-causing agents and may report only selected information to health officials.

Some countries maintain active foodborne disease surveillance systems to determine the burden of foodborne disease more accurately. Such active surveillance systems increase the timeliness of information and provide the baseline incidence, which can be used to measure the effectiveness of control measures. The Foodborne Diseases Active Surveillance Network (FoodNet)[28] in the USA is an example of such a system, based on sentinel sites for determining the burden of foodborne disease. Other networks include OzFoodNet in Australia and the regional network coordinated by the WHO Regional Office for Europe. Unfortunately, most of these systems are not designed to provide rapid or real-time information on foodborne disease outbreaks. Countries need to review their surveillance systems with respect to their capacity to recognize emergencies rapidly. Countries with highly accurate but slow systems should strengthen them to allow rapid detection of food terrorist incidents.

The deliberate contamination of food may be very difficult to recognize, especially if the agent is uncommon and the clinical symptoms are obscure. Linkage of surveillance systems to other related systems might add valuable information for the detection of illness cause by food terrorism. In some cases, deliberate contamination of food may reveal itself through disease clusters in animals. The contamination of animal feed in Belgium with dioxin was detected because animals became sick or died. Linking the veterinary health sector to the surveillance network might thus provide early warning of an incident. Deliberate infection of animals with pathogens of human significance might also be prevented or minimized. Similarly, early detection of deliberate contamination of agricultural products might result in prevention and mitigation of outbreaks in humans.

Improved reporting as a result of effective linkages with health workers, such as pharmacists, and poison information centres could provide information about a potential outbreak in its early stages, or prompt investigation of an undetected disease cluster. Pharmacists could report unusual demand for anti-diarrhoeal agents, anti-emetics or other non-prescription medication that might indicate a food terrorism incident. Industry may receive early warning of food terrorist incidents in the form of inexplicable customers' complaints. Other sources of relevant data

---

[28] Angulo F. J., Voetsch A. C., Vugia D. et al. Determining the burden of human illness from foodborne disease: CDC's emerging infections program foodborne diseases active surveillance network (FoodNet). Vet Clin N Am 1998;14:165–72.

include coroners' reports of unusual deaths, the police forming the link in reporting such data. Absenteeism from schools and the workplace, especially in large industries, can also indicate unusual disease clusters that would trigger investigation.

Routine monitoring for chemical, biological and radionuclear contaminants in food, even if it is not primarily for detection of food safety emergencies, can serve to maintain capacity for identification of an incident and could act as a deterrent to food terrorism. Monitoring provides information on the baseline levels of contaminants in food and can be a good source of information about unusual food contamination during the continuum of farm-to-table. Incidents detected at the stage of food production and processing and at national borders might signal a terrorist attack in the country or elsewhere, thus alerting surveillance systems for early signs of disease clusters and for the need to monitor foods for the suspected agent. Nevertheless, monitoring may not always detect unexpected or unusual contaminants.

3.2.3   *Investigation of suspected food safety emergencies*

3.2.3.1 *Laboratories*

Rapid diagnosis of causative agents during investigation of unexplained disease outbreaks often depends on requesting the appropriate diagnostic laboratory test. Clinicians who become aware of foodborne disease agents must be able to reach the public health sector for advice. The capacity to identify the cause of a disease cluster as an intentional food terrorist act depends on both the circumstances of the case and the sensitivity of the investigative procedures. Rapid response depends on effective links to laboratories with the capacity to identify various foodborne agents, including unusual ones. Such laboratories must have appropriate expertise and analytical methods in place to detect chemical, biological or radionuclear agents in food and in human samples.

3.2.3.2 *Epidemiological investigations*

The objectives of an epidemiological investigation of an outbreak are the same whether they are due to unintentional or covert contamination of food. Identification of the causative agent, the vehicle and the manner of contamination is the most important aspect of the investigation, as it facilitates timely treatment of exposed people and removal of the contaminated food from circulation. Training of epidemiologists may need to be strengthened to include considerations of food and foodborne agents.

Epidemiological investigations should include case definition, case finding, pooling and evaluation of data about potential exposure in various locations. Case–control studies should be conducted to identify specific food vehicles. The investigations should also include collection of laboratory samples, transport and processing of samples, collation of information about sources of contamination and coordination with law enforcement, food safety regulatory authorities and emergency medical response agencies.

3.2.3.3 Investigative tools

Computer-based networks for comparison of bacterial serotypes could enable fast recognition of strains with identical DNA fingerprints, suggesting exposure to a common source and allowing rapid recognition of any connection among geographically dispersed cases[29].

3.3 Preparedness

3.3.1 Principles

The effectiveness of a response depends to a great extent on preparedness plans that are developed and implemented long before any event occurs. Public health preparedness planning for emergency situations has been considered in some detail in various WHO publications and is therefore not discussed in detail in this document[30]. The components of general preparedness plans that enable an effective emergency response include:

- surveillance systems to detect a public health incident;

- implementation of preparedness planning principles;

- testing preparedness plans for effectiveness; and

- assessment of vulnerability to the specific threat or incident:

  - ➤ capacities for investigation and verification of the threat or incident and

  - ➤ linkage of the relevant government agencies and other bodies that will contribute to management of the public health consequences.

Preparedness for response to food terrorist incidents need ton be integrated within existing general plans for emergency response, making maximum use of existing emergency response resources. While food terrorist incidents and threats have special features, it may be unwarranted to form a new, independent response system, as a well-designed public health emergency response system should be able to respond to food terrorist incidents. The principles that underpin the planning process for food safety emergencies need to be consistent with the principles for all emergency response planning. However, the following points are specific to food:

- Planning should consider the ability of the surveillance system to detect food safety emergencies, including those caused deliberately.

- Investigation of a potential outbreak identified by surveillance should include identification of the food and the presence of the responsible agent in the food.

- An incident response should be made concurrently with all the necessary food safety components unless food as a vehicle for the agent can be ruled out.

Preparedness plans should be tested in exercises involving agencies responsible for emergency responses to food terrorism. Any new components should be tested for effective response to

---

[29] Swaminnathan B., Barrett T. J., Hunter S. B. et al. PulseNet: the molecular subtyping network for foodborne bacterial disease surveillance, United States. Emerg Infect Dis 2001;7:382–9.

[30] WHO. Health sector emergency preparedness guide, 1998. www.who.int/disasters.

food terrorism. Evaluation of the results of real incidents and emergency response exercises should be used to identify the need for further resources, refine the roles of various agencies and improve the emergency plans.

The performance of surveillance systems for detecting foodborne disease clusters and epidemiological investigations to identify the food and agent in the food give an indication of the capacity of the system to respond to food terrorism incidents. Timely response to food emergencies, including food terrorism, requires effective linkage of preparedness planning and emergency response systems to all relevant agencies.

If reporting from health care workers and other sources is to be improved, training will be required as a part of preparedness planning. Such training would include increasing capacity to recognize indicators of food safety emergencies, developing reporting modalities and hierarchies and developing the capacity to analyze reports from highly sensitive but nonspecific sources. Suitable laboratory equipment and certification are also important requirements for preparedness. In this regard, it may also be necessary to undertake specialized analytical investigations. Protocols to ensure timely molecular typing and sub-typing of microbiological isolates, prompt transport of isolates to reference laboratories and development of new molecular techniques must all be addressed as part of preparedness planning. Rapid testing for unusual agents, such as dioxin and anthrax, presupposes the existence of specialized laboratories. Member States need to inventory their laboratory capacity at national and regional levels. The priorities for strengthening national laboratory capacity should be commensurate with the threat.

3.3.2 *Assessing vulnerability*

The nature of a response system is based on an assessment of specific threats of deliberate food contamination and their priorities in relation to other public health problems. The priorities are determined as part of an assessment of vulnerability performed before development of preparedness plans for food terrorism. Threats could be ranked from high to low, on the basis of their impact on health and their potential social, economic and political consequences.

Vulnerability is assessed on the basis of the scientific, economic, political and social circumstances of a country, to measure the extent of a threat and to set priorities for resources. Priorities must be set to ensure that the action taken to deal with the threat is commensurate with the severity of the inherent consequences of the threat. The purpose of an assessment of vulnerability is to identify the properties and potential consequences of deliberate contamination of food by harmful agents, to identify relative priorities and to commit national resources in a proportion consistent with these priorities.

Each Member State must assess its own vulnerability, including the effectiveness of the food safety infrastructure, constraints on obtaining chemical, biological or radionuclear agents, motivation for food terrorism, magnitude of the threat associated with a particular agent and mode of delivery, the potential for prevention and the capacity for an effective emergency response. The public health sector must decide on the relative priorities for expenditures, for example, on an oral health programme as opposed to management of food safety emergencies including food terrorist incidents.

An assessment of vulnerability should also include the impact of food terrorism on the national economy. In some Member States, disruption of the export food trade would have disastrous economic consequences, possibly resulting in political destabilization, greater poverty, curtailed development and, ultimately, poorer public health. Vulnerability must be assessed as a multidisciplinary activity, with input from legal, intelligence, medical, scientific, economic and political sectors. National and local circumstances in each Member State need to be considered in the analysis.

Preparedness planning and response systems for food terrorism need to be developed to a level corresponding to the magnitude of the threat assessed. An assessment of vulnerability will also assist national governments in communicating with civil society, allowing a consensus approach for identification of the threat and rationale for the extent of preparedness.

Assessments of vulnerability and other aspects of preparedness should include consideration of the chemical and biological agents and radionuclear materials that could be used to contaminate food. The agents must be assessed for their capacity to cause harm and categorized for priority with regard to resource allocation for preparedness. The CDC's Bioterrorism Preparedness and Response Office has proposed a method for assessing potential biological threats, to guide national public health preparedness and response efforts. This method provides a revisable, reproducible means for standardized evaluation of potential biological threats; however, it focuses on biological agents that cause communicable diseases and does not consider chemical or radionuclear agents or include food as a medium of delivery. Nevertheless, the approach can be modified to accommodate all these elements. The CDC method includes the following aspects:

- the public health impact, on the basis of illness and death, of deliberate exposure to the agent (short- and long-term health effects, severity, vulnerable populations);

- potential for delivery of the agent to large populations on the basis of its characteristics;

- possibility of mass production and distribution of the agent;

- potential person-to-person transmission;

- public perception, as related to fear and potential civil disruption;

- special needs for public health preparedness, including stockpile requirements; and

- need for enhanced surveillance or diagnosis.

Other considerations in an assessment of vulnerability to terrorist incidents might include:

- possibility of obtaining the necessary quantities of an agent (the means to do harm);

- identification of potential terrorists (the will to do harm); and

- the availability and effectiveness of preparedness plans and the capacity for effective response with general preparedness measures (the means to avert harm).

Technical experts in food and food safety should participate in any assessment of vulnerability specific for food terrorism. Information on the toxicology of chemicals and the pathogenicity of microbial agents is a necessary component of such an assessment, together with an assessment of potential exposure, which will determine the potential impact of the agent.

3.4 Response

Response to food terrorism depends on awareness of the possibility of a terrorist act and recognition of the incident as involving food. In many Member States, the overall responsibility for response preparedness rests with an emergency management agency, and the public health aspects are coordinated by the health department. The purpose of preparedness planning is to build a response system that links all the players needed for effective management of an emergency and to develop coordination, communication and integration among local, regional and national resources.

The resources and protocols for a medical response, including rapid transport, supplies, personnel and patient evacuation, are an integral part of communicable disease preparedness, and these have been described elsewhere[31]. Other components that are already included within preparedness planning, such as fire and rescue agencies and specialist response components, have also been described.

3.4.1 Existing emergency response systems

Most Member States have some form of civil defence system to respond to emergencies, such as natural or man-made disasters. The government health sector often coordinates the public health components of these systems. Emergency response systems must be developed within preparedness planning and should be maintained, tested and modified continually in order to adjust to new circumstances. Identification of gaps is an important part of the process and should be undertaken as a matter of priority. The globalization of the food trade means that an inability to respond to a food emergency incident such as food terrorism would have severe consequences on health and trade in many countries.

Public health preparedness and response systems focus mainly on communicable diseases, and most emergency response systems do not yet include consideration of the use of food as a vehicle for terrorist agents. Few countries would be able to respond rapidly and effectively to food terrorism in their current state of development.

In the event of an incident suspected of involving intentional contamination of food, the requirements of the criminal justice system, such as the admissibility in court of any specimens collected need to be taken into account. Preparedness planning should include facilitation of unhampered criminal investigation, which may require adequate legislation, a signed chain of custody for any specimens and effective interaction between emergency response and law enforcement components.

3.4.2 Strengthening existing emergency response systems for food safety

The principles of preparedness planning and emergency response to intentional contamination of food are the same as those for dealing with natural or man-made disasters. Food safety emergencies include either a credible threat or an actual act of deliberate contamination of food. Even if the threat is not credible, public fear must be allayed and action taken to characterize the threat and to locate and prosecute the perpetrators. An emergency response system must allow swift action to assist affected populations and to minimize the adverse consequences of the incident on unaffected populations. The FAO/WHO Codex Alimentarius Commission is

---

[31] Khan A. S., Morse S., Lillibridge S. Public health preparedness for biological terrorism in the USA. Lancet 2000; 356:1179–82.

developing a model food safety emergency plan that provides a useful check list of the principles and phases involved in a model food safety emergency plan.[32]

In strengthening an existing emergency response system to respond to food terrorism, Member States need to:

- identify the necessary components of an emergency response;

- evaluate the effectiveness of the links between existing components for ensuring effective communication and response;

- identify gaps in the existing system;

- link to new components; and

- test the effectiveness and completeness of the emergency response system by simulated exercises or case studies.

Although the structures and agencies that deal with food safety emergencies differ from one country to another, the main players include local and national epidemiologists and laboratories, regulatory agencies for agriculture, health, standards and commerce, and food and health inspectors. Tracing systems to identify and recall contaminated food need to be instituted with government and industry coordination. In cases of food terrorism, the general system should include the law enforcement arm of the government, supported by appropriate legislation. The overriding requirement for an effective response to food safety emergencies predicates links and effective communication among all these players, and their linkage to the existing national preparedness and emergency response system.

3.4.3 *Consequences of a food safety emergency*

An effective public health response to a food terrorist incident will depend on the timeliness and quality of communication among numerous agencies and sectors, including health services, public health authorities at local and national level, clinicians, infectious disease specialists, laboratories, poison information centres, forensic pathologists, other agencies and organizations and the food industry. An effective emergency response must also be tailored to the circumstance and should include links with law enforcement and intelligence agencies, food recall systems, risk assessment specialists and the food industry as well as the more traditional sectors of health care providers, laboratories and emergency services.

Figure 2 illustrates the proposed linkages between existing national alert and response systems and food safety systems to allow effective detection of and response to food terrorist incidents. Improved links with food safety agencies will allow access to relevant information about food and about methods and analytical techniques for testing food and harmful agents. Experts in food safety could assess the risks associated with chemicals and microbiological hazards to ensure that the response is proportional to the risk. Food safety agencies can coordinate food recalls, and generally have well-established links with the food industry to effect rapid removal of unsafe food from circulation. Quarantine and customs agencies have information about food imports necessary for tracing and recall and can undertake rapid seizure of food at the point of

---

[32] FAO/WHO, Proposed Draft Revision to the Codex Guidelines for the Exchange of Information in Food Control Emergency Situations (CAC 19-1995) CX/FICS 02/11/5, September 2002, FAO, Rome

Figure 2. Proposed linkages between existing national alert and
response systems and food safety systems

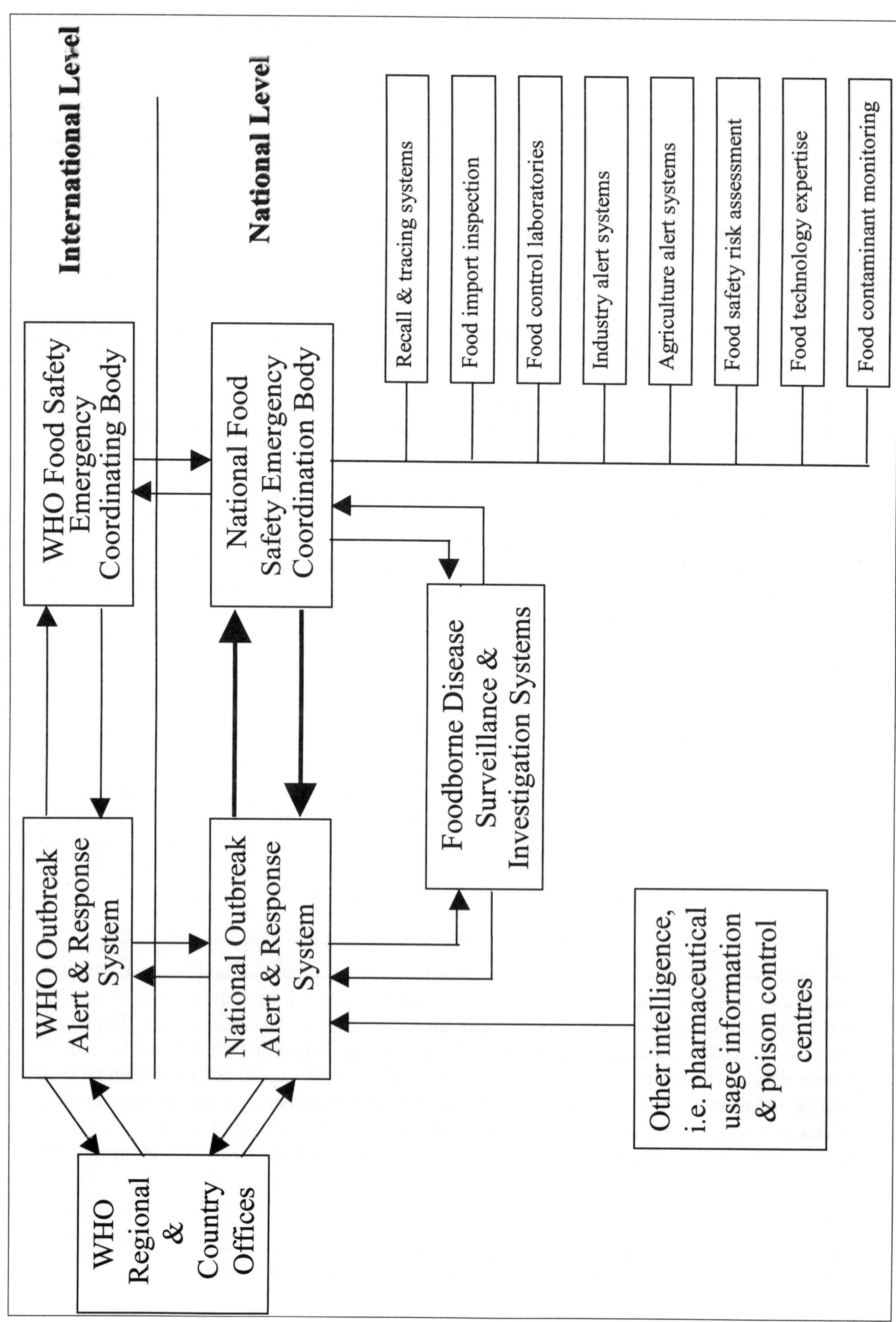

entry. Coverage 'from farm to fork' needs to be incorporated into response planning for food safety emergencies, including food terrorism.

Addition of these links to the existing components of emergency response plans would strengthen the capacity to respond to incidents. Greater awareness of food issues within emergency response is also necessary to achieve rapid, effective mitigation of the consequences of food terrorism.

3.4.4 *Communication*

Swift communication among all the components of an emergency response system is essential and should be an integral part of preparedness planning. The FAO/WHO Codex Alimentarius Commission is revising its Guidelines for Food Safety Exchange of Information in Food Control Emergency Situations (CAC 19-1995) to include information on the management of food safety emergency situations, as well as information on the exchange of information in such situations.[33]

The communication methods used in some Member States to coordinate investigation of geographically dispersed outbreaks might be models for food safety emergencies. Secure Web-based resources would facilitate communication during an emergency response. Because terrorists often seek to create panic and fear in the population, emergency response systems with good communication capacities may even serve to dissuade terrorist attacks.

Industry needs to consider the value of informing government authorities about contamination incidents or hoaxes that may herald a terrorist incident. Industry needs to take into account the social and cultural values and systems in different countries. Such communications need to be consistent and developed in consideration of all stakeholders. Some industry bodies have developed protocols for responding to terrorist threats and have formulated model questions and answers for dealing with the public in such situations.

Communication with the mass media is essential in preparedness planning. Timely press releases and other information must to be ready for the media before unauthorized announcements are released to the public. The availability of trained food safety experts can ensure good communication. Public education and awareness of potential threats contribute to an effective emergency response and should be considered part of preparedness planning. A balanced approach must be taken, providing information without increasing anxiety. Cultural aspects should be considered in communications about threats and incident response, and generalized risk communication approaches may not be applicable. An FAO/WHO publication on risk communication for food safety matters provides some guidance[34]. The Food and Drug Administration in the USA has prepared a list of frequent questions about food safety and terrorism (http://www.cfsan.fda.gov/~dms/fsterrqa.html), which may be a useful guide for communication with consumers on this issue.

Food terrorism hoaxes may overwhelm emergency response systems and cause economic and political disruption. These often follow actual terrorist incidents or threats. Publicity about unsubstantiated threats can be as effective as an actual attack in eroding public confidence in the

---

[33] FAO/WHO, Proposed Draft Revision to the Codex Guidelines for the Exchange of Information in Food Control Emergency Situations (CAC 19-1995), CX/FICS 02/11/5, September 2002, FAO, Rome

[34] FAO/WHO. The application of risk communication to food standards and safety matters. Report of a joint FAO/WHO expert consultation. Food and Nutrition Paper 70. FAO, Rome, 1999.

food supply. In addition to generating panic, such publicity often propagates further hoaxes such as 'copy-cat' impulses which can complicate the emergency response. Hoaxes must therefore be considered in the development of risk communication plans. National and local governments need to review their policies and procedures for managing such situations and, in cooperation with private sector organizations, develop appropriate strategies for communication with the public to manage fear and to control unfounded rumours.

3.4.5 *Launching the response*

The emergency response need to follow the preparedness plan. The responsibilities of lead agencies, whether they be health agencies responding to a medical emergency or law enforcement agencies responding to criminal acts, need to be clearly identified as part of the plan. Emergency responses to food terrorist threats require an unprecedented degree of cooperation among public health and law enforcement agencies of governments, as well as with private sector organizations.

Identification and recall of affected foods are important features of a food safety emergency response. Recall is usually coordinated by food safety agencies with the assistance of the food industry. The food industry is a significant source of information about the quantities of food produced, sources of raw materials and distribution patterns and tracing systems for finished products. This information is necessary for estimating the scale of potential exposure and for removing the affected food from sale. It may also assist in a criminal investigation of a food terrorist incident.

4. The Role of the World Health Organization

4.1   International response to food safety emergencies, including food terrorism

International trade in food, with its rapid, widespread distribution systems, may pose a new international threat to public health, as food that has been contaminated in one country can threaten public health in other countries. Deliberate addition of harmful agents to food can range from large-scale incidents involving bulk food to tampering with individual food items. Widespread media coverage and the resulting panic and fear which can be expected to follow any terrorist incident would lead to increased demand for medical and other emergency services. Measures to address such threats and incidents may be beyond the resources of many Member States and in developing countries may be available only through bilateral or international cooperation. As increasing numbers of Member States may become affected by food terrorist incidents, coordination of international responses has become vital to rapid detecting of incidents, identifying causative agents and foods and responding promptly and effectively to contain and mitigate the effects.

Traditional approaches for the containment of disease outbreaks consist of defensive responses, including securing borders against both the exit and entry of disease, including contaminated food. Such strategies are increasingly being seen as ineffective, failing because of the globalization of the food trade and the unprecedented increase in the movement of people across the globe. The management of threats to public health in the Twenty-first Century, including the threat of food terrorism, requires a combination of early global warning, sensitive surveillance systems, well-tested preparedness plans and rapid emergency responses. Communication and sharing information through internationally coordinated networks will provide timely information for risk management.

4.2   The World Health Organization

WHO is the only international health organization with the primary mandate to protect public health and to provide technical assistance and advice to Member States on all health matters. As an independent, apolitical public body supported by its Member States, WHO has a long standing relationship of trust and privileged access to its Member States. The basic functions of WHO include:

- implementation of the International Health Regulations (IHR);

- coordination of worldwide disease surveillance networks;

- coordination of international responses to communicable diseases;

- assessments of the health risks associated with chemical and biological agents and radionuclear materials; and,

- capacity building functions in food safety and related aspects of public health mainly through its six Regional Offices.

These functions, together with its specific mandate on terrorism from its 196 Member States, place WHO in a unique position to play a key role in:

- coordination of global surveillance for food safety emergencies, including food terrorism;

- facilitation of responses to food emergencies that may be of international significance to human health; and

- provision of technical assistance for national preparedness and response.

Global epidemic surveillance requires an transparent approach and collaboration among many diverse partners. The existing WHO arrangements with national and international partners, including health ministries and scientific institutes as well as various networks and non-governmental organizations, illustrate the success of WHO's coordination of these efforts.

Effective preparedness for food terrorism requires both strengthening of public health surveillance and improved coordination and communication among the sectors responsible for an emergency response. Lack of integrated surveillance, epidemiological and laboratory activities and lack of preparedness planning for emergency response in many developing countries are still significant obstacles to effective detection of and response to threats posed by the deliberate introduction of hazardous agents into food.

4.3   *International Health Regulations (IHR)*

The IHR, agreed by the international community and adopted by WHO in 1969, represent the only regulatory framework for global public health security. IHR can prevent the international spread of infectious diseases by requiring national public health measures that are applicable to travellers and products at the point of entry. While the current IHR require Member States to notify WHO of all cases of cholera, plague and yellow fever, the IHR are undergoing revision to meet the increasingly complex risks of existing and emerging infectious diseases. The revisions proposed include a requirement to notify WHO of all public health emergencies of international concern. In view of the need to contain disease and public health risks at their origin and to minimize international control measures, Member States would be obliged to identify and control events of international public health importance, including infectious and non-infectious diseases as well as high levels of toxins and chemicals in food.

The new IHR will provide guidelines for implementation of requirements for surveillance and response to public health emergencies. The capacities that are to be proposed as essential include rapid detection and reporting of public health emergencies, verification and preliminary control measures and response capacity, including notification to WHO of events or risks of international significance. This would include notification of a need for assistance to contain or control further spread and for travel and traffic restrictions on the free movement of people, conveyances and goods. Information and recommendations developed by WHO would serve as a guide for responses appropriate to the actual health risk. It is anticipated that the revised IHR will be submitted to the World Health Assembly in May 2004.

4.4   Coordination of global outbreak alert and responses

4.4.1   Outbreak alert mechanisms

Under the WHO Programme on Global Alert and Response, WHO has established a mechanism for disease outbreaks that provides accurate and timely information about important disease outbreaks. This information is delivered systematically and rapidly to key professionals in international public health through:

- *Specialized surveillance networks*: WHO has established a number of international networks for specific disease threats, such as FluNet for influenza, RabNet for rabies, Global Salm-Surv for salmonellosis and DengueNet for dengue.

- *Outbreak verification:* Outbreak verification is a new approach to global disease surveillance that aims is to improve control of epidemics by active collection and verification of information on reported outbreaks.

Verification of outbreaks is based on a broad range of sources of information, including the Global Public Health Information Network (GPHIN), which is a Web-based electronic system developed by Health Canada in collaboration with WHO and which scans the Web to identify suspected outbreaks. Suspected outbreaks are followed up with the affected countries to verify the existence of the epidemic, its cause and the measures being taken.

The information is then disseminated via the outbreak verification list to over 900 institutions and key decision-makers in international public health, such as WHO Collaborating Centres, national institutes of public health and the major non-governmental organizations. Since 1996, over 500 outbreak reports have been investigated and the information disseminated when it was found to be of international public health importance. WHO offers assistance in all cases.

4.4.2   Global Outbreak Alert and Response Network

The WHO Global Outbreak Alert and Response Network provides immediate public health assistance for the containment of outbreaks of disease. The Network maintains public health by ensuring coordinated mechanisms for outbreak alert and response. It consists of a technical partnership between institutions and networks and complements existing systems. Its role is to combat the international spread of outbreaks by rapid identification, verification and communication of threats, leading to a coordinated response. It ensures that appropriate technical assistance reaches the affected Member State rapidly, minimizes the health impact of the outbreak and prevents further disease spread.

4.4.3   Outbreak response

WHO responds to requests from Member States for assistance in outbreak management by fielding special teams of experts. Recent examples of outbreaks in which WHO participated directly in the field include: Rift Valley fever in Kenya and Somalia, monkey pox in the Democratic Republic of Congo, avian influenza (H5N1) in Hong Kong (China), Ebola haemorrhagic fever in Gabon, relapsing fever in southern Sudan, influenza in Afghanistan, epidemic dysentery in Sierra Leone, Marburg virus infection in the Democratic Republic of the Congo and Nipah virus in Malaysia.

Active WHO involvement in coordinating epidemic response allows not only provision for immediate needs but also initiation of measures with long term benefits, such as laboratory networks and active surveillance systems. An epidemic represents one of many entry points for greater involvement of WHO in the affected country, to improve epidemic preparedness and response capacity. WHO is working with its partners to improve global, regional and national preparedness for epidemics by providing technical advice and support, including:

- establishing global surveillance and response standards;

- creating networks of partners for preparedness and rapid response (e.g. sub-regional preparedness and response teams in the African Region);

- strengthening laboratory capacity and laboratory networks;

- training in epidemiology; and

- assessment and strengthening of national surveillance systems.

These activities might be focused on one country or be carried out at a regional or international levels. The many broad initiatives for multi-focal recurring needs are exemplified by the cholera task force, which offers immediate support for intervening during epidemics and enhancing preparedness for future events, including stockpiling of essential materials. These activities require a large pool of expertise and are carried out with the assistance of key partner institutions, individuals and donors.

4.5 Strengthening international systems to meet the threat of food terrorism

Member States are requesting leadership, advice and other assistance from WHO to deal with terrorist threats from chemical, biological or radionuclear agents. The existing WHO programmes and coordination activities for surveillance and responsiveness were developed to deal with communicable diseases and may not, in their current form, allow rapid detection of and response to food safety emergencies. Efforts are under way to integrate components into these programmes and activities that would allow rapid detection and effective emergency response to food terrorism.

A holistic approach to surveillance, preparedness and response would include diseases caused by intentional and unintentional contamination of food as well as other media. The review of the IHR anticipates this approach by broadening the regulation framework to provide assessment and response capacity to all public health risks of international importance, including those due to non-infectious agents such as toxins and chemicals. Under the proposed IHR framework, surveillance and response systems and coordination activities carried out by WHO would be strengthened to broaden the current communicable disease focus to detect and respond to food terrorism.

4.5.1 Other existing WHO programmes relevant to food emergencies, including food terrorism

4.5.1.1 Food safety

The Food Safety Department of WHO provides guidance to Member States on matters including establishing and strengthening of food safety infrastructures, including capacities for risk assessment and design of studies of dietary exposure to contaminants that allow national risk assessments. Guidance for establishing and strengthening national food safety infrastructures is provided in a WHO publication[35]. The Food Safety Department is the focal point for WHO collaboration with FAO in the Codex Alimentarius Commission, which implements the Joint FAO/WHO Food Standards Programmes established in 1963. In addition, several other WHO programmes contribute to the overall food safety effort, described below. While these programmes provide many of the elements necessary to strengthen existing alert and response systems to include considerations of food safety emergencies, internal and external links are being strengthened to assure their effective use by Member States.

4.5.1.2 Radionuclear incidents

The WHO Programme on Radiation and Environmental Health coordinates responses to major nuclear and radiation emergencies, which would include deliberate contamination of food with radionuclear agents, with several international agencies including FAO, the International Atomic Energy Agency (IAEA), the Nuclear Energy Agency of the Organisation for Economic Co-operation and Development (OECD), the United Nations Office for the Coordination of Humanitarian Affairs (OCHA) and the World Meteorological Organization (WMO). WHO is a full party to the convention of early notification of a nuclear accident or radiological emergency, the Secretariat of which is at IAEA. Conventions such as this are the main legal instruments for an international framework to facilitate exchange of information and prompt provision of assistance in the event of radiation accidents or other events, such as food terrorism, with the aim of minimizing the health consequences.

4.5.1.3 Chemical incidents and emergencies

The WHO Programme on Chemical Safety serves as the Secretariat for the International Programme on Chemical Safety (IPCS) and provides technical advice and assessments of the risks associated with exposure to certain chemicals. It also promotes harmonization of methods for chemical risk assessment and management and offers guidance for preparedness and response to chemical emergencies. IPCS also promotes the prevention and treatment of poisoning and, through its INTOX database, supports the technical capacity of poison control centres and harmonizes data collection in cases of toxic exposure. IPCS maintains a network of centres and provides technical assistance as requested. It makes available thousands of documents on chemical safety and the sound management of chemicals on a CD-ROM (INCHEM) and via an Internet site www.inchem.org, for Member States and individuals. IPCS has also developed an emergency response network to deal with chemical accidents and spills.

4.5.1.4 Monitoring and exposure assessment of chemicals in food

The WHO Global Environmental Monitoring System/Food Contamination Monitoring and Assessment Programme (GEMS/Food) provides information on concentrations of chemical contaminants in food, their contribution to total human exposure and their significance for public health and trade. GEMS/Food provides baselines of chemical contaminants in food against which may be used to assess deliberate contamination. The Programme is an important component of the global risk assessment of chemicals in food and provides exposure assessments which form part of the basis for setting national and international food safety standards. GEMS/Food maintains a network of WHO Collaborating Centres, national focal points and

---

[35] WHO. Guidelines for strengthening a national food safety programme. WHO/FNU/FOS/96.2. Geneva, 1996.

participating institutions located in over 70 countries. It maintains links with international organizations such as FAO, IAEA, the United Nations Environment Programme (UNEP) and nongovernmental organizations such as the International Union of Food Science and Technology (IUFoST) and the International Union of Pure and Applied Chemistry.

4.5.1.5 Risk assessment of chemical and microbiological agents

The Joint FAO/WHO Expert Committee on Food Additives (JECFA) and the Joint FAO/WHO Meetings on Pesticide Residues (JMPR) assess the risks associated with chemicals in food, for use by Member States and by the Codex Alimentarius Commission. WHO, in collaboration with FAO, has initiated risk assessment of microbiological agents in food through the Joint FAO/WHO Expert Meetings on Microbiological Risk Assessment (JEMRA). The WHO Food Safety Department can thus coordinate expert advice on specific chemical and microbiological threats in food. Risk assessment and technical advice are vital tools in assessing the threat represented by food terrorism and in ensuring that the resources committed for preparedness plans and emergency responses at the international level are proportional to the threat.

4.5.1.6 Foodborne disease surveillance

Many Member States maintain surveillance programmes to detect foodborne disease outbreaks, as outlined in the previous chapter. In collaboration with the WHO Food Safety Department, the WHO Programme on Emerging Public Health Risks including Drug Resistance has embarked on a programme to coordinate global foodborne disease surveillance networks, to complement the Global Public Health Information Network and strengthen countries' capacity to detect foodborne illness of international significance including those that may be due to food terrorists.

4.5.1.7 WHO Guidelines for Drinking-water Quality

Drinking-water and water used as an ingredient in food processing and cooking can be important in food terrorism. First published in 1984, the WHO Guidelines have been used as a basis for setting international and national standards to ensure the safety of water supplies. Under the WHO Water, Sanitation and Health Programme, guideline values for a large number of water constituents and contaminants, including certain potential terrorist agents, have been set.

4.5.2   Other international organizations relevant to food safety

WHO collaborates closely with FAO and the International Office of Epizootics (OIE) on food safety matters. While WHO has the mandate to address aspects of human health as they pertain to food, FAO primarily addresses agricultural production and food sufficiency issues. For example, the FAO Plant Protection Service address issues of plant health and quarantine matters. FAO is also developing an electronic information exchange mechanism (Biosecurity Portal) which will provide a single access point for national and international information on food quality and safety, plant health and animal health. The International Office of Epizootics is concerned primarily with animal health and quarantine issues. Links between these and other international organizations result in increased capacity to detect and investigate foodborne emergency of international significance.

4.5.3 Coordination and strengthening of international strategies and activities that address food safety emergencies, including deliberate contamination of food

The existing strategies and activities of the WHO Food Safety Department are being effectively linked with other WHO programmes to coordinate detection of and response to foodborne diseases. The resulting linked system would provide a stronger international coordination of outbreak alert and response for illness associated with foodborne pathogens but would also address food terrorist threats.

Expansion of current WHO risk assessment activities and training programmes to include food safety emergencies such as food terrorism would assist Member Sates, especially developing countries, to build capacity to respond to food safety emergencies. With the support of its Member States and the donor community, WHO can strengthen its efforts to assist Member States in responding to this potentially devastating public health threat. The Executive Board of the WHO adopted a resolution on 17 January 2002 in which response to terrorist acts with chemical and biological agents was identified as a clear priority for WHO and its Member States. The Fifty-fifth World Health Assembly in May 2002 requested WHO to provide tools and support for Member States to strengthen their national health systems, notably with regard to emergency preparedness and response plans. For further information on the WHO food terrorism activities, readers are directed to contact the WHO Representative in their country or to contact directly the WHO Food Safety Department.

Specific Measures for Consideration by the Food Industry

This Appendix outlines specific measures that could be considered by the food industry. Smaller, less developed companies will clearly not be able to implement all of them. Essentially, the risk for food contamination by terrorists can be minimized by creating awareness among employees that the threats must be taken seriously and by reducing the opportunities for unnoticed contamination by restricting access to production lines and products. Some Web sites that give more detailed information are listed at the end of this Appendix.

1.   *Risk awareness*

Review your business and company procedures, physical facility, processes, shipping and distribution systems. Identify and list all areas where you may be vulnerable to a terrorist attack. Identify and outline control measures for each of these areas.

Identify any neighbouring facilities that could contaminate the environment if there was an accident, including nuclear power stations, enrichment centres and waste storage facilities.

Know the origin of all your raw materials and be aware of the possibilities for contamination during their harvesting, production and transport.

Train all your employees in food safety and security procedures. Extend the training to all new employees. Provide periodic reminders of the importance of security procedures.

Train and hold employees accountable for recognizing and reporting suspicious activity and suspect persons, signs of possible tampering with products and equipment and other unusual circumstances.

Provide instructions for employees who may be threatened or who suspect product tampering by other employees.

2.   *General security*

Assign responsibility for food security to a qualified person. Identify a food security management team and critical decision-makers.

Conduct daily security checks of your premises for signs of tampering with products or equipment, other unusual circumstances or areas that may be vulnerable to tampering.

Check all toilets, maintenance closets, personal lockers and storage areas regularly for concealed packages or other anomalies.

Eliminate potential hiding places within your facility where an intentional contaminant could be placed temporarily before introduction.

Maintain an up-to-date floor plan showing access points; keep it in a secure location, and give it to local fire officials.

Provide adequate lighting both inside and outside the facility, and provide emergency lighting.

Use metal or metal-clad doors whenever possible.

Establish procedures for after-hours or night-shift security.

Account for tools and utensils such as knives used by employees on a daily basis.

Account for all keys to the establishment.

Emergency alert systems must be fully operational and tested. The location of controls, escape routes and emergency exits should be clearly marked.

Immediately investigate all reports of unusual or suspicious activity, including those in the immediate vicinity of the facility. Document all the investigations and report all problems to the local authorities.

Watch for unusual behaviour by (new) employees or workers, e.g. staying unusually late after the end of a shift or working day, arriving unusually early, consulting files or areas outside their field of responsibility, removing documents from the facility or asking questions on sensitive subjects.

In the event of suspected sabotage or terrorism, contact the local police and indicate the concern. When possible, <u>do not move or touch</u> the affected product, equipment or material; cordon off the area to limit access; move any employees who were in the vicinity or may have been affected to a secure area away from other people.

Develop a clearly documented, well-rehearsed product recall plan. Have written plans for deciding upon and evaluating the scope of a recall. The plan must include the immediate recall of the product from trade and consumer channels when tampering and/or contamination is suspected. Ensure that all product sold can be traced to the relevant trade customer.

Keep the details of food security procedures confidential.

2.1   *Mail handling*

Handle mail in a separate room or facility, well away from food handling and processing areas.

Train mail handlers to recognize and handle suspicious pieces of mail.

2.2   *Data security*

Restrict access to computer process control systems for food products and critical data systems to those with appropriate clearance. Protect passwords and use network firewalls and effective, current virus detection systems.

Ensure that all recipes, production data and analytical results are properly backed up (electronic or hard copies at another location, updated regularly), at a frequency that should be reviewed for adequacy.

Challenge the computer security system regularly and audit routinely to ensure that security procedures are in place.

Remove computer access rights from employees immediately after voluntary or involuntary termination.

2.3 *Threats*

Report any threats or aberrant behaviour to the proper authorities.

3. *Emergency procedures*

Create an emergency response team and develop an action plan to be followed in the event of tampering, terrorist activity or any other type of emergency. Test your plan to make sure that it works and then make any necessary adjustments, employee training or equipment purchases.

Identify local, state and central government contacts. Have a list of names and numbers of primary and secondary contacts in all regulatory agencies. Have internal, fire and police emergency phone numbers available.

Prepare and test procedures for emergency evacuation of the facility.

Train employees in emergency procedures for dealing with various situations (such as a bomb threat, fire, flooding or chemical spill). Include this training as part of the orientation programme for new employees.

Provide information on emergency procedures and evacuation routes to all visitors and contract workers.

Establish procedures with local community emergency personnel to assure proper access to the facility during an emergency, while preventing public access.

Set up procedures to deal with onlookers or media representatives who might be present during an emergency.

4. *Hazardous materials*

Review the hazardous materials stored on the facility and reduce them to the absolute minimum necessary for operations, both in number and quantity. These may include sanitation chemicals, pesticides, laboratory reagents, toxin standards and pathogen cultures.

Inspect chemicals on receipt and verify their authenticity.

Ensure that all hazardous materials are stored in a locked area away from food handling processing and food areas. Ensure that all hazardous materials are clearly and correctly labelled.

Have safety sheets available for all hazardous chemicals stored on site.

Control access to any laboratory where hazardous chemicals and live cultures of pathogenic bacteria are stored. Restrict access to specially designated persons.

Restrict laboratory materials to the laboratory, unless required for activities such as sampling.

Establish clear procedures for the control and disposal of pathogenic cultures if these are handled in the laboratory.

Maintain an accurate inventory of all hazardous materials. Verify it on a daily basis and immediately investigate missing stock or other irregularities.

For water-treatment chemicals, set up a foolproof system for ensuring correct identity and dosage. Reconcile the amounts used with remaining stock at least weekly.

5.   *Employees*

Establish procedures for screening applicants before employment. At the least, verify the immigration status, work references, addresses and phone numbers supplied on the application form. In certain cases, other protocols, such as drug testing and criminal background checks, might be implemented.

Apply the same, uniform screening procedures to employees already working at the facility and to all seasonal, temporary and contract workers. Request that the same screening procedures be applied by outside hiring agencies, if used.

Do not allow new employees to work before such verification checks have been made.

Have a system for positive employee identification, such as photo identification badges with an identification number.

Place new employees on day shift with supervision during probation.

Maintain an updated list of employees with open or restricted access to the facility.

Maintain a roster of employees working on any given day, by shift. Know who is and who should be on the premises and where they should be located. Distribute the roster to supervisors.

5.1   *Personal items*

Restrict the personal items allowed in the establishment.

Prohibit certain types of personal items (e.g. lunch containers, bags, thermoses and drink containers) in food handling areas. Put procedures in place for enforcing these rules.

Provide lockable storage facilities for employees' personal items. Establish authority and procedures to permit inspection of these lockers.

When the company provides clothing or protective gear for work in the facility, prohibit such garments from being taken home by the employee.

Do not allow employees and visitors to bring cameras into the facility.

6.   *Access*

Clearly define the outer boundary of the facility, within which access should be limited or controlled. Control access to this restricted area, by use of guards, access cards, etc. Erect fencing or other barriers to prevent unauthorized entry

Identify areas within the restricted boundary that are of greater concern than others, e.g. water storage tanks and outside storage tanks for cleaning chemicals, coolants and ingredients. Limit or monitor access to these areas. Ensure that the frequency of monitoring is sufficient to detect any abnormality. Clearly define responsibility for monitoring and controlling these areas. Give the relevant individuals the authority to take immediate action if there are signs of a problem.

Secure all bulk storage tanks with locks, seals, sensors or warning devices.

Control entrance to the facility by employees reporting for work, and control the departure of employees leaving the facility during normal working hours. Institute special controls for employees entering or leaving the facility outside normal hours of work.

Ensure that all the normal routes for personnel entry to or exit from the facility are monitored or controlled. Where feasible and legal, consider reducing the number of entry and exit points. Maintain the legally required number of emergency exits and ensure that these cannot be used as entry points (e.g. self-locking doors that can be opened only from the inside).

Assess any other possibilities for access, such as equipment room entrances, air ducts, windows, roof openings and vent openings. Seal or provide with locks.

Have procedures in place to restrict access to the facility by terminated employees.

Require positive identification of all visitors, including contract workers, supplier representatives, customers, auditors and data entry and computer support staff. Provide badges to such visitors and collect them when they leave the facility.

Restrict access of visitors and guests, including friends and relations of employees and applicants for employment. Restrict these visitors to non-production areas unless they are accompanied by an authorized plant representative. Exercise particular caution with unannounced visitors.

Provide special waiting areas and rest rooms for drivers delivering or collecting goods. Do not allow drivers to enter restricted areas.

Define sensitive or critical areas within the facility where personnel access and movement should be further restricted. These should include raw material and finished product warehouses, chemical storage facilities and access to central controls for air handling, water systems, electricity and gas supplies. Clearly mark and secure these restricted areas. Allow only designated employees to enter.

As far as possible, limit access only to those areas necessary for the employee's work. Consider methods or devices, such as colour-coded uniforms or coded badges, to make it obvious when employees move to areas of the facility other than those where they normally work.

Restrict access by contractors and their employees to those areas of the plant relevant to their work.

Periodically reassess levels of access for all employees.

Keep vehicle and bicycle parking areas well separated from the production and storage areas, water facilities and fuel tanks. Assess whether access to employee parking areas should be restricted or monitored (e.g. use of stickers, access cards).

Monitor all incoming and outgoing vehicles (both private and commercial) for unusual cargo or activity.

7. Suppliers

Know your suppliers and purchase only from contracted suppliers, as far as possible. Be aware of the special risks of products bought on the open market.

Make all suppliers aware of food security issues and insist that they implement appropriate controls. For agricultural produce, they must be especially aware of the potential risks of contamination on the farm and be vigilant with regard to unusual traffic on the road or in the air and other circumstances.

Include in purchasing contracts a requirement that suppliers must provide commodity codes and expiration dates, with written explanations in case of recalls and other food safety actions.

Request and inspect records of products transported previously in tankers, railcars and shipping containers. Include this requirement in purchasing and transport contracts.

8. Raw and packaging materials

All lots of ingredients and supplies must be uniquely identified and traceable to the supplier and a specific manufacturing or processing facility. Compare transport documents (bills of lading, delivery slips) with the orders made by your company

Insist on seals or other tamper-evident packaging features, whenever possible, for ingredients and chemicals used in food processing or for other uses such as cleaning or water treatment.

Inspect all incoming materials (ingredients, packaging, labels, supplies) and their shipping containers for signs of tampering, counterfeiting, contamination or other anomalies. Refuse any packages or containers with signs of tampering (damaged, leaking or resealed packages) or counterfeiting (evidence of unauthorized relabelling or repackaging).

Verify the identity and authenticity of all ingredients and chemicals by cross-checking the labels against the shipping documents and by applying simple tests.

Maintain all incoming goods on hold (under quarantine) until formally released for use based on satisfactory inspection and verification results.

8.1 Water

Identify all sources of water used in the facility (both potable and non-potable sources) and implement appropriate security measures for each source. Secure access to all water wells, storage tanks and handling facilities, to prevent unauthorized entry.

If a municipal water supply is used, ensure that predetermined procedures are in place for prompt two-way communication with responsible officials in the event of any abnormalities in the supply.

Develop procedures to assure the integrity and security of the water used, including restricted access to the water system, with only designated employees allowed in the area, and use of tamper-evident connectors and valves.

Inspect potable and non-potable water lines in food processing areas periodically for possible tampering.

Test potable water regularly. Verify that pH, conductivity, active chlorine (where relevant), odour, appearance (colour, turbidity), taste and total plate count are within the normal ranges.

9.   *Storage areas and warehouses*

Maintain controlled access to all product and ingredient storage areas. Restrict access to storage areas to designated employees.

Pay special attention to off-site storage facilities (e.g. controlled temperature rooms) used for holding products or ingredients before processing. Ensure that they are configured and monitored to handle and hold products securely.

Keep labels in a secure area to prevent theft or misuse. Destroy all outdated product labels.

Keep an accurate inventory of ingredients, packaging, labels and finished products (including location). The system must allow detection of unexplained additions to or withdrawals from existing stock. Investigate missing stock or other irregularities and report any problems to the local authorities.

Perform random inspections of storage facilities to ensure that the security programmes are appropriate and effective.

10.   *Processing areas*

Identify any areas where employees mix or batch products or ingredients by themselves without supervision. Put controls in place to prevent tampering by an employee.

Restrict access to areas in which large amounts of product are exposed, e.g. vats, kettles, tanks, chillers and coolers.

Identify points where clandestine access to ingredients or products is possible. Evaluate whether these points can be minimized or monitored.

Evaluate potential clandestine use of equipment for the purpose of introducing a contaminant.

Supervise contract workers, maintenance and sanitation staff, cleaning crews and pest controllers who would be able to contaminate a product or an ingredient intentionally.

Provide special instruction and/or training for contractors who work in sensitive areas.

10.1 *Processing systems*

Ensure that all processing systems, including automatic control systems, are secure. Identify the persons authorized to access the control systems and to modify the processing parameters.

Verify the integrity of the packaging of all ingredients before use.

Set up procedures to be followed in the event of intentional contamination during the production process, including mixing of processed and unprocessed products (e.g. retort bypass). These procedures must ensure timely identification, segregation and security of all intermediate and finished products.

Ensure complete traceability, from raw materials to finished products and from finished products to raw and packaging materials.

Verify the use of sensitive ingredients (e.g. spices, additives, vitamins and mineral salts) at the end of each day. Reconcile the remaining stock with the actual use, preferably by someone other than the employee who weighed out or added the ingredient.

As far as possible, do not allow returned goods to enter the facility. If this is unavoidable, examine the returned goods for evidence of tampering before salvage or reuse. Keep records of the destination of all returned goods.

11. *Transport of ingredients and processed products*

Use reputable, reliable transport companies and confirm that they have appropriate controls in place.

Require transport companies to conduct background checks on drivers and other employees with access to the product.

Require that the vehicles used for transport of raw material and finished products or other material used in food processing are never left without supervision or made accessible to outsiders. Investigate any unexplained delay or deviation in the schedule of deliveries.

For incoming shipments, require locked and sealed vehicles, containers and/or railcars. Require the seal numbers to be identified on shipping documents. Verify the shipping seals with shipping papers before unloading. Refuse delivery if the seal is broken (unless the driver or his company gives a valid reason). Investigate shipping documents with suspicious alterations.

Have procedures in place for trucks entering the facility boundaries. Require advance notification from the supplier of all deliveries. Notification should include pertinent details about the shipment, including the name of the driver. Verify truck deliveries against a roster of scheduled deliveries. Unscheduled deliveries should be held outside the facility premises, if possible, pending verification of the shipper and cargo.

Supervise off-loading of incoming ingredients, packaging and labels.

All outgoing shipments should be sealed with tamper-evident, numbered seals that are listed on the shipping documents.

Secure loading docks to avoid unverified or unauthorized deliveries.

Tankers bringing milk from farms and collection centres should be sealed at both the milk inlet and the milk outlet between collection and delivery.

Introduce special procedures for off-hour deliveries; require the presence of an authorized person to verify and receive the shipment.

All trailers on the premises must be locked and sealed at all times when not being loaded or unloaded.

Websites

http://www.who.int/fsf/ (Food Safety, World Health Organization)

http://www.who.int/emc/deliberate_epi.html (Communicable Disease Surveillance and Response, World Health Organization)

http://www.who.int/disasters (Emergency and Humanitarian Action, World Health Organization)

http://www.cfsan.fda.gov/~dms/fsterr.html (Food and Drug Administration, Center for Food Safety and Applied Nutrition, USA)

http://www.foodsafety.gov/~fsg/bioterr.html (Food and Drug Administration, Center for Food Safety and Applied Nutrition, USA)

http://www.inspection.gc.ca/english/ops/secur/secure.shtml (Canadian Food Inspection Agency)

http://www.nfpa-food.org/members/science/101101foodsecurity.asp (National Food processors Association, USA)

http://www.fsis.usda.gov/oa/topics/securityguide.htm (Food Safety and Inspection Service)

Terrorist Threats to Food: Guidance for Establishing and Strengthening Prevention and Response Systems

Addendum

(Insert, page 34)

4.5.1.8 *WHO European Region Task Force on Biological, Chemical and Nuclear Emergencies*

The WHO European Region has established an interim Task Force to better coordinate national and regional activities in response to the threat to civilian populations from deliberate use of biological and chemical agents and nuclear materials. This includes development of networks for emergency preparedness and response, for technical experts and institutions and for national focal points. Activities include assessment of preparedness in Member States, development of a regional plan of action for strengthening capacities, coordination with relevant other regional and international organizations, and provision of advice on technical matters, communication and resource mobilization. The Task Force is chaired by the Humanitarian Assistance and Emergency Preparedness Programme of the WHO Regional Office for Europe based in Copenhagen and supported by relevant technical programmes, including food safety.

(Replacement Text, page 34)

4.5.2 *Other international organizations relevant to food safety*

WHO collaborates closely with FAO and the Office international des épizooties (OIE) on food safety matters. Links between these and other international organizations result in increased capacity to detect and investigate foodborne emergencies of international significance. While WHO has the mandate to address aspects of human health as they pertain to food, FAO addresses agricultural production and food security, including food quality and safety issues. WHO has many links with the food safety aspects of FAO programmes. These programmes are implemented in the context of food security – to ensure the access of all to sufficient, safe and nutritious food. In meeting this mandate, FAO provides advice to member governments (including food producers, food industry and consumers) on application of food safety management systems, and effective national controls to prevent food contamination. More broadly, FAO provides support to agriculture and fishing communities to improve production and to better the condition of rural populations. This combination of assuring a safe and nutritious food for all, while supporting the agriculture and fisheries sectors makes a suitable entry point for responsible action along the food chain. In addition to food safety, the FAO Plant Protection Service addresses plant health and quarantine matters while animal health matters are the concern of the Animal Production and Health Division.

Recent FAO initiatives include the development of the biosecurity programme and the convening of a series of meetings to discuss the framework of biosecurity as a tool for national governments to manage risks associated with food and agriculture. In addition to food safety, this includes the sectors of plant life and health, animal life and health and biosafety. An international Internet-based portal for the exchange of information on official regulatory requirements covering the different sectors of biosecurity is under active development by FAO in collaboration with other relevant agencies.

The OIE is concerned primarily with animal health and quarantine issues. Due to the increasing demand of consumers in improving food safety worldwide, the OIE has identified the need to expand its normative and scientific activities into "animal production food safety" and to work with other relevant organizations in addressing and preventing the "production to consumption" foodborne hazards of animal products (meat, milk, eggs, honey etc.).